Kidney Cleanse

A Complete Guide to Optimizing Kidney Function

(Perfect Manual to How Natural Herbs Can Be Used to Cure Kidney Disease)

Clyde Santiago

Published By **Kate Sanders**

Clyde Santiago

All Rights Reserved

*Kidney Cleanse: A Complete Guide to Optimizing
Kidney Function (Perfect Manual to How Natural
Herbs Can Be Used to Cure Kidney Disease)*

ISBN 978-1-7386412-4-6

No part of this guidebook shall be reproduced in any form without permission in writing from the publisher except in the case of brief quotations embodied in critical articles or reviews.

Legal & Disclaimer

The information contained in this book is not designed to replace or take the place of any form of medicine or professional medical advice. The information in this book has been provided for educational & entertainment purposes only.

The information contained in this book has been compiled from sources deemed reliable, and it is accurate to the best of the Author's knowledge; however, the Author cannot guarantee its accuracy and validity and cannot be held liable for any errors or omissions. Changes are periodically made to this book. You must consult your doctor or get professional medical advice before using any of the suggested remedies, techniques, or information in this book.

Table Of Contents

Chapter 1: The Main Causes and Risk Factors

Welcome to the primary financial disaster of "Renew Your Kidneys, Restore Your Life: A Holistic Approach to Kidney Health and Wellness." In this bankruptcy, we are capable of dive deep into facts the roots of kidney disorder, exploring the number one motives and hazard elements that make a contribution to this condition By dropping moderate on those essential components, we intention to empower you with the information and gadget essential to transform your kidney fitness and renew your existence.

Kidney illness is a conventional state of affairs that affects tens of thousands and thousands global, however it stays alarmingly underestimated and misunderstood. This bankruptcy serves as a complete manual, permitting you to understand the underlying motives that would reason this illness. We will discover various factors which include immoderate blood stress, diabetes, medicinal tablets, pollutants, and their ability impact on your kidneys.

However, this financial disaster is going beyond actually listing the causes of kidney sickness. We may also delve into the intricacies of risk factors that warrant close to interest. By figuring out those elements in your non-public life, you can advantage precious perception into what may additionally moreover cause kidney ailment. Whether or no longer it is a circle of relatives records of the state of affairs, smoking conduct, or weight issues, records the risks can permit proactive measures in the direction of prevention and early intervention.

It is essential to famend the placement that persistent kidney illness plays within the improvement of kidney disorder. By familiarizing yourself with the complexities of this situation, you can benefit a higher understanding of its behavior and capability headaches. Understanding how poorly controlled medical situations, collectively with diabetes and excessive blood strain, drastically increase the chance of growing this situation will inspire you to prioritize your state-of-the-art health if you want to protect your kidney characteristic.

Furthermore, we are able to shed moderate on the gradual improvement of persistent kidney disease, emphasizing the significance of early detection and intervention. Armed with this statistics, you'll be able to actively pick out any caution signs and symptoms and signs or signs and signs and signs and symptoms, prompting well timed motion to prevent in addition damage.

The facts contained in this economic wreck is not high-quality enlightening but serves as a vital tool for taking manage of your kidney health and ability reversal of kidney sickness. By leveraging this facts, you will be prepared to make informed choices approximately your way of life, clinical manage, and widespread properly-being.

Join us in unraveling the roots of kidney illness and set yourself on a path within the course of a life of colourful kidney health and fitness. Together, we're capable of navigate this journey of renewal, sharing the understanding that stems from severa sources of information and indigenous recovery practices. Embrace this bankruptcy because the first stepping stone within the direction of renewed electricity and a restored experience of well-being.

Why Understanding the Causes and Risk Factors of Kidney Disease is Crucial for Your Health

The solar commenced out to set over the small metropolis, painting the sky with colourful sunglasses of crimson and orange. Mary sat by myself on her porch, her mind heavy with fear. The medical doctor's terms replayed in her head like a damaged document: chronic kidney sickness.

Mary had typically been a strong woman, a person who confronted lifestyles's annoying conditions head-on. But this evaluation had struck her at her center, leaving her feeling inclined and scared. She refused to accept an entire life of dependence on medicines and dialysis. There needed to be a few different manner.

As she sat there, enveloped by using using using the serenity of her surroundings, her eyes wandered to the lovely garden blooming in her out of doors. Each flower stood tall and resilient, symbolizing the energy she longed to regain. That's even as she remembered paying attention to approximately the indigenous recovery concepts from an antique buddy who had professional remarkable effects.

With newfound willpower, Mary launched into a adventure of self-discovery. She delved into the complicated international of pioneering holistic strategies to kidney renewal, devouring books and filling her kitchen with an array of culinary herbs, sourced right away from mom nature herself.

It wasn't an clean direction. Mary faced limitless doubters, skeptics who shook their heads and advised her it modified into all nonsense. But she persevered, buoyed through stories of indigenous healers who had unlocked the secrets and techniques and strategies of self-recovery.

Day after day, Mary practiced deceleration techniques, embracing moments of stillness and meditation amidst the chaos of her daily regular. The waves of calm that washed over her brought renewed desire and strength, a spark that ignited her perseverance.

Slowly however surely, the threat factors that after loomed over her started out to expend. The manner of lifestyles choices that had driven her kidneys to the threshold of collapse have been now modified with nourishing options. Cigarettes have been traded for walks inside the crisp morning air, and immoderate portions gave manner to carefully crafted food full of nutrient-rich additives.

The hours became days, and the days into months. Mary's strength of mind to her adventure become unwavering. And because the seasons handed and the colorful flora in her lawn bloomed anew, so too did her power.

Her most modern visit to the doctor have become met with astonishment. Improvements were obvious, and her kidney characteristic had taken a large flip for the better. The as quickly as skeptical clinical specialists now marveled at her perseverance and its ensuing outcomes.

Mary's eyes sparkled with newfound desire as she lower returned domestic, feeling the load of the area carry off her shoulders. Through information the roots of kidney sickness and embracing a holistic approach to recuperation, she had defied all odds and carved a route to renewal.

As Mary sat on her porch once more, a sly smile completed on her lips. She had conquered the battle that had threatened to engulf her existence, proving the power of self-recuperation and customized self-control. The sun dipped below the horizon, casting long shadows all through the garden, however Mary knew that a brand new sunrise awaited her each morning – a testament to the resilience of the human spirit and the importance of embracing a holistic technique to kidney health.

And with each passing day, Mary persevered to release the secrets and strategies of self-restoration, nurturing her body, mind, and soul, as she weaved her high-quality story into the tapestry of possibility.

Understanding the Roots of Kidney Disease: The Main Causes and Risk Factors

High blood strain, diabetes, and high-quality medicinal drugs or pollution are the precept reasons of kidney sickness. In this chapter, you may find out how those elements can make contributions to kidney damage and why it is crucial to understand them for early detection and prevention. By gaining belief into the motives of kidney disease, you will be higher ready to make important manner of existence changes and discover remedy options that address the ones underlying troubles.

Firstly, allow's delve into the relationship between excessive blood strain and kidney damage. High blood strain, additionally referred to as excessive blood stress, can strain the blood vessels to your kidneys, impairing their capability to filter waste and additional fluid correctly. Over time, this pressure can purpose kidney damage and in the long run chronic kidney contamination. It is essential to manipulate your blood strain via regular tracking, medication if prescribed by using manner of your healthcare issuer, and adopting a coronary coronary heart-healthy way of lifestyles that includes a balanced food regimen and everyday workout.

Next, we are capable of discover the relationship among diabetes and kidney disorder. Diabetes is a situation characterized through excessive blood sugar ranges, and it can cause damage to the tiny blood vessels inside the kidneys. This harm impairs the kidneys' filtration characteristic, main to the buildup of waste and fluids within the body. To prevent or manage diabetes-associated kidney sickness, it's miles important to maintain tight manage over your blood sugar levels thru medicinal drug, nutritional adjustments, everyday physical interest, and monitoring your kidney function frequently.

Certain medications and pollution can also have detrimental consequences on kidney function. Some medicinal tablets, together with nonsteroidal anti-inflammatory tablets (NSAIDs) like ibuprofen and naproxen, and tremendous antibiotics, can damage the kidneys whilst used excessively or for prolonged intervals. Additionally, exposure to effective pollution, together with heavy metals or commercial enterprise chemical materials, can make contributions to kidney damage. It is vital to be aware of the capability dangers related to drug treatments and pollutants and speak any issues along side your healthcare employer. They can provide steering on secure utilization and help you perceive any crucial adjustments to protect your kidney health.

Understanding the ones causes of kidney disorder is important for early detection and prevention. By recognizing the threat factors and making critical manner of existence adjustments, you can lessen the hazard of developing kidney disease or gradual its development if already identified. For example, adopting a diet plan that includes some of fruits, greens, complete grains, lean proteins, and restrained sodium and sugar intake can manual kidney fitness. Additionally, everyday exercising, retaining a wholesome weight, and fending off smoking are all life-style factors that might honestly effect kidney characteristic.

In summary, immoderate blood stress, diabetes, nice medicinal pills, and pollution can contribute to kidney sickness. Understanding those reasons allows for early detection and prevention. By managing blood stress, controlling diabetes, being aware of remedy utilization, and minimizing exposure to pollutants, you may shield your kidneys. Making way of life adjustments collectively with adopting a healthy eating regimen, wearing out regular exercising, retaining a healthy weight, and keeping off smoking can also extensively decorate kidney health. Remember, it is within your energy to take control of your kidney health and save you or manipulate kidney illness.

Chapter 2: The Main Causes and Risk Factors

Risk elements for kidney disorder consist of a circle of relative's records of the situation, smoking, and weight problems. These factors can substantially growth your chances of growing kidney sickness and data their impact is essential for taking proactive measures to reduce your hazard.

1. The Impact of Genetics and Family History on Kidney Disease Risk

Your circle of relatives data performs a huge feature in identifying your risk of developing kidney disorder. If you've got have been given near accomplice and kids, which includes dad and mom or siblings, who've been identified with kidney infection, you're much more likely to expand the state of affairs as well. This is due to the fact high quality genetic factors can predispose people to kidney problems.

While you can not trade your genetic make-up, being privy to your family facts permits you to be proactive in dealing with your kidney health. Regular screenings and test-u.S.A.Come to be even more essential if kidney contamination runs in your circle of relatives. By staying vigilant and working carefully together with your healthcare employer, you could capture any signs of kidney sickness early and take suitable motion.

2. How Smoking Can Contribute to Kidney Damage

Smoking isn't always most effective risky in your lungs and coronary coronary heart however moreover poses a huge danger on your kidneys. The chemicals determined in cigarettes can motive damage to the blood vessels in the kidneys, main to decreased blood go together with the glide and impaired kidney characteristic through the years.

Additionally, smoking will growth your blood strain, further straining your kidneys and developing the risk of kidney sickness.

To defend your kidneys, it's far essential to surrender smoking or avoid tobacco products altogether. Quitting smoking is a tough manner, but there are resources to be had to guide you on your journey. Speak to your healthcare employer approximately cessation packages or help groups that can help you prevent smoking and enhance your ordinary kidney fitness.

3. The Connection Between Obesity and Kidney Disease

Obesity is a diagnosed hazard issue for various fitness situations, which includes kidney ailment. Excess weight locations greater strain at the kidneys, leading to increased blood stress and capacity harm to the filtering gadgets of the kidneys. Furthermore, obesity is regularly related to other health troubles like diabetes and excessive blood pressure, each of which could in addition exacerbate kidney problems.

Maintaining a healthful weight via regular exercising and a balanced weight loss program is critical for lowering your threat of kidney illness. By adopting a lifestyle that consists of physical interest and nutritious consuming conduct, you can't handiest control your weight however additionally guide best kidney feature. Focus on eating masses of culmination, vegetables, whole grains, lean proteins, and healthy fats to nourish your frame and promote kidney fitness.

four. The Importance of Recognizing These Risk Factors and Taking Proactive Measures

Recognizing the danger elements associated with kidney sickness is the first step inside the direction of protective your kidney fitness. By being privy to your family information, keeping off smoking, and keeping a wholesome weight, you may extensively reduce your hazard of growing kidney infection. Proactive measures like regular test-ups, screenings, and lifestyle modifications are critical for early detection and prevention.

five. Strategies for Reducing the Risk Associated with Each Factor

To lessen your danger of kidney illness, maintain in thoughts implementing the following techniques:

Stay knowledgeable about your own family facts and communicate it together together with your healthcare company.

Seek useful resource and assets to surrender smoking and shield your lungs and kidneys.

Maintain a wholesome weight via everyday exercising and a balanced diet.

Limit your intake of processed elements, sugar, and threatening fats.

Stay hydrated via eating an proper enough quantity of water during the day.

Manage underlying scientific situations together with diabetes and hypertension thru right remedy and monitoring.

By taking these proactive steps, you could appreciably decorate your kidney health and reduce your possibilities of developing kidney ailment. It's important to hold in mind that small modifications can also moreover have a massive impact, and thru prioritizing your fitness, you're setting your self on a path in the direction of renewed energy and nicely-being.

Understanding the Role of Chronic Kidney Disease in the Development of Kidney Disease: Preventing Complications

Chronic kidney contamination (CKD) is a time period that refers back to the gradual lack of kidney characteristic over time. It is a revolutionary situation that could result in similarly harm if left untreated. In this section, we are able to discover the definition and improvement of CKD, the significance of early detection and intervention, functionality complications that might rise up from untreated CKD, and strategies for stopping or mitigating the ones headaches.

To begin, let's outline chronic kidney disease. CKD is characterised through manner of the slow and irreversible decline in kidney function, critical to the construct-up of waste merchandise and fluids within the body. This decline is regularly measured using the glomerular filtration price (GFR), which shows how properly the kidneys are filtering waste from the blood. As the GFR decreases, the kidney's capability to do away with waste diminishes, ensuing within the accumulation of pollution and fluid imbalances.

The development of CKD is a regarding element of this case. Without proper control, CKD can result in in addition damage and complications. As cited in advance, CKD is a modern circumstance, because of this that it worsens over time if not addressed. The decline in kidney feature may be categorised into stages, with stage 1 being the mildest and level 5 representing give up-degree renal illness (ESRD). Each degree shows a lower in the kidney's functionality to clear out waste and modify physical capabilities.

Early detection and intervention play a important function in managing CKD correctly. By figuring out and addressing CKD in its early ranges, you can gradual down the improvement and probable maintain kidney function. Regular screenings and tests, which includes blood and urine tests, can help hit upon abnormalities in kidney characteristic earlier than symptoms and signs get up. Early intervention may additionally additionally comprise way of life adjustments, which includes dietary modifications, coping with blood stress, and controlling blood sugar tiers, depending at the underlying causes of CKD.

Neglecting the control of persistent kidney disorder can bring about numerous complications. These headaches ought to have an impact on unique factors of the body and fashionable fitness. Untreated CKD can result in cardiovascular problems, which incorporates immoderate blood pressure, coronary heart illness, and stroke. The accumulation of waste products also can reason bone loss, anemia, and weakened immune feature. Additionally, CKD will boom the chance of growing precise situations, at the side of kidney infections or kidney stones.

Preventing or mitigating complications is a important detail of coping with chronic kidney contamination. Proper control includes regular tracking of kidney characteristic through laboratory exams and check-u.S.With healthcare experts. Lifestyle changes, including maintaining a wholesome weight-reduction plan low in sodium and phosphorus, dealing with blood pressure and blood sugar ranges, and engaging in everyday bodily activity, can also assist reduce the risk of headaches.

In summary, information the characteristic of chronic kidney sickness inside the improvement of kidney sickness is critical for preventing headaches. Chronic kidney disease is a contemporary state of affairs that requires early detection and intervention to gradual down its improvement. Neglecting right manage can motive headaches that have an effect on numerous elements of fitness. By enforcing techniques collectively with ordinary screenings, life-style modifications, and ongoing monitoring, you can mitigate the chance of complications and decorate your everyday kidney health. In the subsequent sections, we are able to delve deeper into particular techniques and interventions to aid your kidney health adventure.

Chapter 3: Hypertension on Kidney Health

When it involves kidney health, it's miles crucial to recognize the big feature that poorly managed medical conditions, which incorporates diabetes and excessive blood pressure (excessive blood stress), can play in developing the risk of developing kidney sickness. In this segment, we're capable of delve into how those situations can impact kidney function and discover the importance of tracking and controlling them to lessen the threat of kidney contamination. We may additionally provide an outline of remedy alternatives and life-style changes that would assist manage diabetes and hypertension, while highlighting the viable headaches that might upward push up if those situations are ignored of manipulate.

Uncontrolled diabetes may have destructive outcomes on kidney feature.

When blood sugar stages are always high, it is able to harm the small blood vessels in the kidneys, impairing their capability to smooth out waste materials from the body correctly. Over time, this could result in a state of affairs known as diabetic nephropathy; it really is a not unusual purpose of chronic kidney illness. It is vital for people with diabetes to cautiously monitor their blood sugar stages, adhere to their prescribed medicinal drugs, and take a look at a wholesome weight-reduction plan to help hold strong blood sugar tiers and save you or slow down the improvement of kidney damage.

Hypertension, or excessive blood stress, is a few different most vital contributor to kidney illness. The kidneys play a crucial role in regulating blood stress by means of filtering excess fluid and sodium from the body. However, whilst blood stress remains continuously extended, it is able to strain the sensitive blood vessels in the kidneys and reduce their efficiency. This pressure can ultimately motive kidney damage or even kidney failure. Managing immoderate blood stress through lifestyle adjustments, on the facet of adopting a low-sodium diet, conducting normal bodily activity, and taking prescribed medicinal drugs, can appreciably lessen the danger of kidney headaches.

Monitoring and controlling diabetes and excessive blood pressure is important for lowering the chance of kidney illness. Regular check-u.S.A.With healthcare corporations are vital to evaluate blood sugar levels, blood pressure readings, and not unusual kidney characteristic. By carefully adhering to the endorsed remedy plans, humans can decrease the prolonged-term impact of these conditions on their kidneys. It is essential to word that everybody's treatment plan can also furthermore variety primarily based mostly on man or woman health needs and medical steering. Therefore, it is always encouraged to examine the advice of healthcare professionals.

In addition to scientific interventions, extremely good way of lifestyles adjustments also can assist manage diabetes and high blood strain, therefore decreasing the chance of kidney disease. For humans with diabetes, adopting a balanced weight loss program rich in give up result, vegetables, complete grains, and lean proteins can aid in blood sugar manage. Regular bodily interest can also enhance insulin sensitivity and contribute to normal cardiovascular fitness. Likewise, for human beings with immoderate blood stress, decreasing sodium intake, growing potassium-wealthy elements, and appealing in regular workout can help in maintaining healthy blood stress tiers.

If left out of control, both diabetes and high blood pressure can cause intense complications beyond kidney illness. Uncontrolled diabetes can increase the chance of cardiovascular problems, nerve damage, imaginative and prescient loss, or maybe lower limb amputations. Similarly, untreated excessive blood stress can make contributions to coronary coronary heart disorder, stroke, and precise vascular issues. Therefore, taking proactive measures to control these conditions now not best improves kidney fitness however also enhances primary properly-being and reduces the danger of numerous related fitness troubles.

In summary, know-how the effect of poorly controlled clinical situations, such as diabetes and excessive blood stress, on kidney health is vital for preventing the development of kidney ailment. By carefully monitoring and dealing with the ones conditions, human beings can reduce the threat of kidney headaches and decorate ordinary fitness consequences. Combining scientific interventions, collectively with medicinal tablets and normal check-ups, with way of lifestyles modifications like adopting a healthful diet and attractive in physical activity, can play a huge characteristic in retaining sturdy blood sugar tiers, handling blood pressure, and helping most appropriate kidney characteristic. Taking manage of these situations is essential for unlocking the secrets and techniques of self-healing and nurturing vibrant kidney fitness.

Understanding the Stages of Chronic Kidney Disease and the Importance of Early Intervention

Chronic kidney ailment (CKD) is a present day-day scenario that may have immoderate effects if left untreated. It is crucial to apprehend the levels of CKD and the functionality dangers related to its development. By understanding how CKD develops and the importance of early detection and treatment, you can take proactive steps to gradual down its progression and guard your kidney health.

Stages of Chronic Kidney Disease:

CKD is normally classified into 5 stages based definitely mostly on the extent of kidney harm and the decline in kidney feature. Each degree represents a one-of-a-kind diploma of severity, with stage 1 being the mildest and diploma five indicating give up-degree renal illness (ESRD). Let's find out the ones tiers in greater detail:

1. Stage 1: Kidney damage with everyday or expanded filtration charge.

During this stage, there can be proof of kidney harm, inclusive of protein or blood in the urine, however the kidneys are though functioning normally. The number one precedence at this degree is to emerge as privy to the underlying cause of kidney damage and implement measures to save you in addition development.

2. Stage 2: Mildly decreased filtration rate.

In level 2, there's a slight decrease in kidney characteristic, but it is able to no longer however cause extremely good symptoms. Regular monitoring and manner of life modifications are important to gradual down the development of CKD.

3. Stage three: Moderately decreased filtration fee.

At this level, kidney function is appreciably impaired, and symptoms may also moreover start to occur. Fatigue, fluid retention, and modifications in urination styles are common signs and symptoms. It is crucial to paintings intently together together with your healthcare employer to govern CKD and prevent further complications.

4. Stage four: Severely decreased filtration rate.

Stage four suggests a intense decline in kidney function, with signs and signs and symptoms and signs turning into greater stated. Patients can also experience anemia, bone troubles, and elevated vulnerability to infections. Medical intervention, which includes nutritional adjustments and medication manage, is important to hold balance and gradual down the development of CKD.

5. Stage five: End-degree renal sickness (ESRD).

This is the maximum advanced diploma of CKD, wherein kidney function is significantly impaired, and dialysis or a kidney transplant becomes important for survival. It is important to prevent CKD from progressing to this stage via seeking out early intervention and closely following encouraged treatment plans.

Consequences of Untreated Chronic Kidney Disease:

If left untreated, persistent kidney ailment can result in excessive complications that can impact not best your kidney health but moreover your familiar nicely-being. Some capability outcomes embody:

1. Cardiovascular Disease:

CKD will boom the chance of developing cardiovascular issues including coronary coronary heart assaults, strokes, and excessive blood stress. The decline in kidney characteristic can disrupt the frame's stability of fluids and electrolytes, essential to an stepped forward strain on the coronary coronary heart.

2. Anemia:

As kidney feature declines, the manufacturing of pink blood cells decreases, resulting in anemia. This can cause fatigue, inclined factor, and problem concentrating.

3. Bone Disorders:

Impaired kidney characteristic can disrupt the steadiness of calcium and phosphate within the frame, leading to weakened bones and an expanded hazard of fractures.

Importance of Early Detection and Prompt Treatment:

Early detection and intervention are important in coping with chronic kidney illness correctly. By identifying CKD in its early tiers, healthcare companies can enforce appropriate measures to sluggish down its improvement and limit the hazard of complications.

Monitoring Techniques and Tests for Assessing Kidney Function:

To determine kidney feature and show display screen the development of CKD, numerous tests and techniques are applied. These can also additionally encompass blood exams to degree creatinine and estimate glomerular filtration price (GFR), urine checks to find protein or blood inside the urine, and imaging research like ultrasound or CT scans to assess the form and period of the kidneys.

Interventions and Lifestyle Modifications to Slow the Progression of CKD:

There are several interventions and lifestyle changes that may help slow down the development of CKD:

1. Medication Management:

Your healthcare company might also additionally moreover prescribe medicinal drugs to govern blood pressure, manipulate diabetes, reduce proteinuria (immoderate protein within the urine), or deal with unique underlying situations contributing to CKD.

2. Dietary Changes:

A wholesome weight loss plan performs a essential characteristic in handling CKD. Limiting sodium, phosphorus, and potassium intake, controlling protein intake, and keeping a balanced food plan rich in fruits, greens, and entire grains can help maintain kidney characteristic.

3. Blood Sugar Control:

If you have diabetes, it is essential to keep your blood sugar ranges beneath manipulate. This can be accomplished thru medication, dietary adjustments, everyday exercise, and everyday tracking.

By understanding the levels of CKD, the functionality effects of untreated sickness, the importance of early detection and activate remedy, further to the monitoring strategies and interventions available, you can take an energetic function in defensive your kidney fitness. Remember, early intervention is essential to slowing down the improvement of persistent kidney illness and preserving maximum reliable kidney feature.

Understanding the Importance of Early Detection and Intervention in Kidney Disease Management

Early detection and intervention play a pivotal role in handling and doubtlessly reversing kidney disease. By prioritizing ordinary screenings or exams, you may proactively turn out to be aware of any signs and symptoms and symptoms of kidney disease and take right away motion to save you similarly damage. In this phase, we are able to explore why early detection is vital, how it is able to assist control or perhaps contrary kidney sickness, and the diverse remedy alternatives and lifestyle modifications that may useful resource kidney health.

Routine screenings and assessments are crucial for early detection of kidney sickness. Regular take a look at-u.S.With your healthcare business enterprise allow for the tracking of key signs and symptoms together with blood stress, blood glucose levels, and urine albumin tiers. These exams can flag capability problems in advance than symptoms and signs take place, supplying an possibility for well timed intervention. By staying vigilant approximately these screenings, you empower yourself with valuable information approximately your kidney fitness.

Early intervention is vital in correctly coping with and in all likelihood reversing kidney sickness. When detected at an early stage, steps can be taken to sluggish down the development of kidney damage and maintain renal feature. This often consists of implementing way of existence adjustments and incorporating specific remedy alternatives or restoration techniques.

Treatment alternatives within the early levels of kidney sickness recognition on addressing the underlying reasons and managing related conditions. For instance, if immoderate blood strain is identified as a contributing aspect, remedy and manner of existence modifications can assist control it and reduce the strain at the kidneys. Similarly, if diabetes is observed to be a hassle, preserving most appropriate blood sugar levels thru dietary adjustments and medicine can assist save you similarly kidney harm. The creator emphasizes the significance of working cautiously together along with your healthcare company to expand a custom designed treatment plan tailor-made to your particular needs.

In addition to clinical interventions, adopting positive way of existence modifications and self-care practices can extensively help your kidney fitness. The author highlights the significance of maintaining a balanced and nutritious weight loss plan, proscribing sodium and brought sugars, and staying hydrated. Implementing everyday exercise physical activities, dealing with pressure ranges, and operating in the direction of mindfulness and relaxation techniques also are recommended techniques for promoting kidney health and ordinary properly-being.

Success memories and studies studies offer encouraging evidence of the impact that early intervention can also have on kidney illness development. Numerous folks that were proactive approximately their kidney fitness and sought early medical hobby have experienced superior kidney feature or maybe reversal of the illness. These fulfillment memories characteristic notion and beautify the importance of taking motion on the earliest feasible stage.

Research studies have moreover established the blessings of early intervention in slowing down the improvement of kidney illness. By addressing underlying reasons, managing related situations, and implementing manner of lifestyles modifications, individuals were capable of keep renal feature and maintain a higher nice of existence. This scientific evidence further reinforces the significance of early detection and intervention.

In conclusion, early detection and intervention are essential in efficaciously dealing with and in all likelihood reversing kidney disease. Routine screenings, collectively with blood stress and urine albumin assessments, permit the identification of kidney ailment in its early stages. By right away addressing underlying reasons, coping with related situations, and incorporating manner of lifestyles modifications, you can drastically assist your kidney fitness and in all likelihood gradual down illness improvement. The strength to take control of your kidney fitness lies for your palms, and by means of prioritizing early detection and intervention, you may unlock the secrets of self-recuperation and nurture a life of colorful kidney fitness and health.

2. The Power of Indigenous Healing: How Traditional Practices Can Transform Your Kidney Health

Welcome to Chapter 2 of "The Power of Indigenous Healing: How Traditional Practices Can Transform Your Kidney Health." In this economic catastrophe, we're capable of delve into the wealth of expertise and knowledge that indigenous healing practices want to provide in revitalizing our kidney health.

For centuries, indigenous cultures round the arena have trusted those traditional practices to cope with various ailments, along with kidney illnesses. These ancient restoration strategies offer us with a totally particular mindset on the reasons and imbalances that contribute to kidney health issues, providing a holistic method to restoration that encompasses the physical, emotional, and spiritual components of our being.

One of the essential mind of indigenous healing is the popularity that our our bodies aren't isolated structures but are deeply interconnected with nature and the universe. By embracing this interconnectedness, we can faucet into the herbal remedies that our ancestors have used for generations. Medicinal herbs and plants play a incredible function in indigenous restoration, assisting kidney characteristic and promoting regular fitness.

Furthermore, indigenous recovery offers us an possibility to reconnect with the awareness of our ancestors, guiding us on a path towards the renewal of our kidneys. By turning to those conventional practices, we open ourselves to powerful healing energies that have been handed down through generations, enriching and enlivening our our our bodies and spirits.

In this financial ruin, we're able to discover the different factors of indigenous restoration techniques which could advantage every our physical and religious well-being. Integrating mindfulness, meditation, and rituals into our ordinary lives, we are able to embark on a transformative adventure towards harmonizing our body, thoughts, and spirit. With an emphasis on holistic recovery, we are able to discover how those practices provide us now not best consolation from bodily signs however moreover a deeper knowledge and connection with ourselves.

Chapter 4: The Importance Of Embracing Indigenous Healing

Amidst the big expanse of the Amazon rainforest, a ray of daytime broke through the dense canopy, illuminating a serene clearing. In the coronary coronary heart of this lush inexperienced sanctuary stood Maria, a woman whose weary eyes contemplated the toll that years of kidney illness had taken on her.

Maria had commonly possessed an unwavering spirit, but her failing kidneys threatened to extinguish the mild internal her. Countless visits to docs and specialists had yielded little effects, leaving her feeling helpless and annoyed. The traditional treatments she had persisted excellent furnished quick consolation, regularly leaving within the returned of a route of harsh side consequences. But Maria refused to actually take delivery of a life of dialysis and infinite tablets she knew there needed to be some other manner.

Her journey led her to a remote village nestled deep within the rainforest, in which the records of historic recovery practices embraced her like an extended-lost pal. The indigenous healers welcomed her with open arms, sensing her desperation and craving for a one-of-a-type technique. They shared testimonies exceeded down thru generations, tales of colourful health finished thru complex combos of culinary herbs and particular deceleration strategies.

Embracing each word spoken thru the use of the healers, Maria placed a cutting-edge experience of want. The route laid out in advance than her modified into illuminated with shimmering opportunities, not best for her kidneys but for her ordinary nicely being. It wasn't quite lots treating the physical symptoms and signs and symptoms; it have turn out to be approximately nurturing her emotional and non secular self, harmonizing her complete being.

As Maria delved deeper into the recuperation practices, a profound transformation commenced to unfold. She covered medicinal herbs and flora into her food regimen, witnessing firsthand their robust capability to assist kidney function. The nourishment she supplied her frame become now not restricted to pills and injections but bloomed forth as a sensitive symphony of flavors and aromas from nature's very personal bounty.

Each morning, due to the fact the mist hugged the boundaries of the wooded location, Maria engaged in mindfulness and meditation, a sacred communicate collectively along with her frame that instilled a experience of tranquility and properly-being. And in the historical rituals of the indigenous healers, she placed a connection to some element far greater than herself. Through dance and ceremony, she tapped into effective energies that surged via her veins, igniting a renewed feel of strength.

As months exceeded, the tremors of hopelessness that once shackled Maria loosened their grip. With every passing day, her kidney function improved, carving new pathways inside the route of recuperation and renewal. The pain and fatigue that had grow to be her regular partners progressively diminished, great remnants of reminiscence.

Through the power of indigenous restoration, Maria unlocked the gates to her non-public self-recovery capability. She wasn't truely restoring her kidneys; she turn out to be reclaiming her existence, resurrecting the desires and aspirations she had believed had been forever out of attain.

Maria's journey serves as a testomony to the transformative functionality of embracing conventional practices to nourish our kidneys and rejuvenate our souls. It reminds us that deep in the forests of our ancestors lie keys to unlocking our private healing powers. By tapping into the understanding of the indigenous healers and incorporating their profound information into our lives, we can also chart a route to renewed power and embrace the boundless treasures existence has to provide.

The Power of Indigenous Healing: How Traditional Practices Can Transform Your Kidney Health

Indigenous restoration practices have a rich statistics that spans centuries and were applied to treat diverse health situations, together with kidney sickness. These therapeutic strategies are deeply rooted in conventional cultures and have been exceeded down via generations, supplying profound insights into the healing ability of the human frame. By exploring the understanding of indigenous recovery, you may find out a holistic method to transforming your kidney fitness.

Throughout data, indigenous restoration practices have established their effectiveness in treating kidney ailment. Ancient civilizations, collectively with the Aztecs and the Chinese, evolved complex systems of recuperation that centered on restoring stability and concord inside the body. These practices recognized the interconnectedness of all additives of health and understood that imbalances inside the emotional, religious, and bodily geographical regions may additionally want to take place as kidney health problems.

Traditional treatments applied in indigenous recovery for kidney health encompass a large range of strategies, which include the use of medicinal herbs and plant life, rituals, and ceremonies. Herbal remedies have lengthy been seemed as powerful device for assisting kidney feature and selling commonplace fitness. Time-examined herbs together with nettle leaf and dandelion root have proven large advantages in nourishing the kidneys and assisting their renewal.

What devices indigenous healing practices aside from conventional scientific treatments for kidney infection is their holistic approach. While present day medication frequently focuses definitely on addressing the physical symptoms, traditional practices apprehend that real healing consists of the thoughts, frame, and spirit. By exploring the underlying motives and imbalances that make contributions to kidney health issues, indigenous recuperation offers a completely particular perspective which can result in transformative outcomes.

In indigenous healing, the emphasis goes beyond just treating the physical symptoms of kidney sickness. These practices delve deeper into the emotional and religious factors of the character, acknowledging the profound have an impact on those elements have on common well-being. By addressing emotional and spiritual imbalances related to kidney sickness, conventional healers manual the character's regular fitness and facilitate a extra complete recuperation method.

One of the hallmarks of indigenous restoration is the usage of natural remedies derived from medicinal herbs and plant life. These treatments play a crucial feature in helping kidney function and promoting common fitness. Traditional healers have large understanding of the medicinal homes of numerous herbs and plants and the manner to put together and administer them effectively. By incorporating these natural remedies into your kidney restoration journey, you could harness the strength of nature to assist your body's innate healing mechanisms.

By embracing traditional practices, you have got the possibility to tap into the historical consciousness of your ancestors and get right of entry to powerful recuperation energies for kidney renewal. Indigenous recuperation recognizes the significance of ancestral connection and the statistics that can be acquired from reconnecting together with your cultural ancient beyond. Through strategies collectively with rituals and ceremonies, you could channel effective recovery energies into your kidneys, nurturing their power and selling desired fitness.

Mindfulness, meditation, and rituals additionally play a big function in indigenous healing practices for kidney health. These techniques are finished to promote common nicely-being and harmonize the frame, mind, and spirit. By incorporating mindfulness and meditation into your every day exercising, you may domesticate a deeper reference to your body and boom a heightened cognizance of your kidney health. Rituals and ceremonies associated with kidney recuperation offer a sacred place for intentional recuperation and might deepen your reference to your inner self.

Incorporating the strength of indigenous restoration practices into your kidney restoration journey offers a totally unique and transformative technique to improving your kidney health. By embracing the expertise of historic cultures, you could faucet into the holistic nature of recuperation and loose up the secrets and techniques of self-restoration. With every step you take in this course, you circulate inside the route of living a lifestyles of colorful kidney health and common fitness.

The Power of Indigenous Healing: How Traditional Practices Can Transform Your Kidney Health

Understanding the holistic approach of traditional practices:

In our current-day society, we frequently interest completely on the bodily additives of health almost about treating kidney disorder. However, traditional indigenous restoration practices provide a unique perspective, emphasizing the holistic method to properly-being. These practices apprehend that our emotional, non secular, and bodily states are interconnected and must be addressed together for proper restoration to get up.

Exploring the relationship among emotional, spiritual, and physical imbalances in kidney health:

Traditional healers understand that imbalances in our emotional and non secular properly-being can take area as physical signs and symptoms and signs and signs and symptoms, along with kidney sickness. For example, in excessive great indigenous perception structures, emotions which includes fear, anger, and resentment are believed to have an effect on the kidneys straight away. By addressing those emotional imbalances, we're capable of promote kidney fitness and preferred properly-being.

How traditional practices pick out out out and address root reasons of kidney disorder:

Unlike traditional medicinal drug, which often focuses on treating signs and signs, conventional practices are looking for to perceive and cope with the idea motives of kidney infection. These root causes can range from person to man or woman, however they'll encompass lively imbalances, ancestral connections, or unresolved emotional traumas. By statistics and addressing the ones underlying motives, traditional healers goal to repair balance and sell kidney healing.

three. A Holistic Approach to Kidney Renewal: Combining Nutrition, Mindfulness, and Herbal Remedies

Welcome to Chapter three of "Understanding the Roots of Kidney

Disease and Embracing Renewal." In this financial destroy, we delve deep into the paintings of kidney renewal with the aid of the usage of exploring a holistic method that encompasses nutrients, mindfulness, and natural remedies.

When it involves recovery our our our bodies, it's miles essential to take a multifaceted approach. In this bankruptcy, we are capable of find out the effective blessings of blending the ones 3 pillars — nutrients, mindfulness, and herbal remedies — to help the renewal of your kidneys and optimize your essential well-being.

First and crucial, we are capable of find out the critical function of vitamins in selling kidney fitness and facilitating the way of renewal. Learn approximately nutrient-wealthy factors that can offer your body with the important elements it dreams for last kidney feature and rejuvenation. Discover how the proper diet plan may also need to make all the difference not surely in addressing present kidney troubles, however in stopping future headaches as properly.

Mindfulness, a workout often associated with intellectual and emotional well being, performs a great role in kidney renewal. We will delve into severa mindfulness techniques that characteristic effective machine for lowering pressure, selling rest, and revitalizing your kidneys. By incorporating those techniques into your every day routine, you may create an surroundings conducive to the renewal and strength of your kidneys.

Additionally, we are capable of discover the mysteries of herbal treatments particularly tailored for kidney fitness. Discover natures hidden treasures — herbs that have been traditionally used for hundreds of years to manual kidney characteristic and promote recovery. Learn about their unique houses and functionality benefits as we find out the secrets and techniques and strategies of indigenous recovery.

As we retain, the bankruptcy addresses the concept of synergy — how the mixture of vitamins, mindfulness, and herbal remedies can paintings in harmony to decorate the renewal of your kidneys. By expertise and embracing this holistic technique, you may unencumber the real potential of your frame's innate restoration abilties.

But implementation is as crucial as knowledge itself. Therefore, we provide techniques and insights on a manner to encompass the ones practices into your day by day ordinary and lead them to a sustainable manner of life. By reworking the ones strategies into each day behavior, you offer yourself the lasting gift of colourful kidney fitness and easy health.

Lastly, we emphasize the importance of thinking about the rules and capacity interactions of natural treatments supporting herbal healing calls for warning and proper steerage. We strongly inspire consulting with a healthcare professional earlier than embarking on any new remedy recurring to make sure protection and suitability to your unique times.

We invite you to embark in this informational adventure, empowering yourself with the information and gear critical for embracing a holistic technique to kidney renewal. Let us embark together towards the direction of colorful kidney health and properly being like in no manner in advances that.

Chapter 5: The Power of Integration

The solar slowly raised over the mist-protected mountains, casting warmness, golden glow throughout the quiet village. Nestled amongst fields of colorful inexperienced, there stood a humble wooden cabin, belonging to Maria, a woman whose existence were weighed down with the beneficial useful resource of the weight of kidney disorder for a ways too lengthy.

Maria had spent countless days teetering getting ready to melancholy, her as soon as colorful spirit dwindled by using the constant fatigue and pain that coursed thru her body. She had attempted every traditional remedy available, enduring the detail outcomes and praying for a glimmer of preference. But as her circumstance persisted to go to pot, preference appeared like a much off reminiscence, fading just like the sun shades of a sun-bleached portray.

One fateful day, as Maria sat weakly through her kitchen table, she stumbled upon a worn, dirt-protected ebook nestled amongst piles of forgotten papers. Its name leapt off the web page, "Renewing Kidneys, Nurturing Life: The Indigenous Healing Principles". At that 2d, some thing deep inner Maria stirred, an intuitive pull toward a tremendous direction, as although the whispers of her ancestors were guiding her inside the route of profound restoration.

Within its pages, the writer illuminated the significance of a holistic technique to kidney renewal, one that embraced the synergy of nutrients, mindfulness, and herbal treatments. Maria's weary eyes grew brighter as she delved into the wealthy tapestry of statistics unraveling before her. For the number one time in years, she felt a flicker of want blooming interior her chest.

Determined to understand onto this lifeline, Maria set out on a adventure to nourish her kidneys, igniting a hearth inner her spirit. She started out incorporating nutrient-rich meals into her weight-reduction plan colourful end result, leafy greens, and whole grains crammed her plate, infusing her body with the critical constructing blocks needed for rejuvenation.

Mindfulness have become the anchor amidst Maria's stormy seas. With each breath, she permit go of the weight of pressure and anxiety, coming across the power of relaxation in helping her kidney renewal. Through meditation and slight movement, Maria discovered a sanctuary inside herself, growing a fertile floor for her internal healing to flourish.

As Maria embraced the expertise of the indigenous recuperation practices tucked in the ebook's pages, she embarked on a voyage to discover the energy of herbal treatments. She determined out of culinary herbs that now not best infused her meals with flavor however moreover advanced kidney fitness cleaning dandelion root, soothing marshmallow leaf, and antioxidant-wealthy nettle leaf. With each whiff and sip, Maria may additionally want to almost flavor the revitalization coursing through her veins.

The days turn out to be weeks, and weeks into months, as Maria diligently followed the direction of holistic kitchen alchemy — blending nutrients, mindfulness, and natural treatments into her each day ordinary. Slowly, she felt the shackles of kidney disorder loosening, as her energy surged, and her as quickly as-dimmed spark started to blaze first-rate all once more.

Through the pain and tears shed, Maria overcame the constraints that had limited her for an extended way too long. It wasn't continuously clean, however now she knew that she held the important thing to her private recuperation in her capable fingers. Armed with those transformative practices, she bloomed like a wasteland flower after a thunderstorm exceeded, radiantly and unapologetically alive.

Driven via the profound transformation she professional, Maria reveled in a renewed revel in of gratitude and electricity. She released right into a task to percentage her tale, empowering others who were led off beam thru conventional medical conventions. With every word she spoke, every coronary coronary coronary heart she touched, Maria breathed existence into the historical art work of holistic kidney renewal.

In the depths of Maria's battle lay a treasure trove of facts that might all of the time exchange her existence. Through nutrients, mindfulness, and herbal remedies, she unlocked the secrets and techniques and techniques of self-recovery, paving the manner for a existence of renewed energy. With dedication blazing like a wildfire internal her eyes, Maria have turn out to be a beacon of desire, illuminating the direction for all who yearned for kidney renewal and nurturing lifestyles.

And so it changed into, Maria's story whispered through the winds, all the time etching their fact deep in the hearts of these searching out a holistic approach to kidney renewal.

A Holistic Approach to Kidney Renewal: Combining Nutrition, Mindfulness, and Herbal Remedies

In this financial ruin, we can delve into the significance of incorporating nutrient-wealthy meals into your weight loss program to manual kidney health and promote renewal. Your kidneys play a vital function in filtering waste products and pollutants from your body, so it's miles critical to offer them with the nourishment they want to characteristic optimally. By data the characteristic of key nutrients in kidney health and incorporating precise additives into your diet, you can take proactive steps towards enhancing your kidney feature and general properly-being.

Antioxidants, nutrients, and minerals are essential for keeping kidney fitness. Antioxidants protect your cells from damage because of dangerous free radicals, whilst vitamins and minerals

71

guide numerous bodily features. Incorporating a whole lot of nutrient-wealthy food into your weight loss program can make certain that you are presenting your body with the essential building blocks for kidney renewal.

Leafy veggies, which include spinach and kale, are super sources of antioxidants, vitamins A and C, and minerals like magnesium and potassium. These vitamins assist lessen contamination and useful resource kidney function. Berries, together with blueberries and strawberries, are packed with antioxidants and are referred to for his or her anti-inflammatory homes. They furthermore consist of vitamin C, fiber, and phytonutrients that sell kidney health.

Fish, specifically fatty fish like salmon and mackerel, is wealthy in omega-3 fatty acids, that have been tested to reduce contamination and protect against kidney harm. These fish moreover provide amazing protein, vital for preserving muscle tissues and helping kidney feature. Other protein property, collectively with lean poultry, eggs, and legumes, may be covered into your food to ensure an top enough intake.

Meal planning plays a vast feature in prioritizing kidney fitness. Structuring your meals round nutrient-rich meals will assist you to meet your nutritional goals. Consider including some of vegetables, quit give up end result, complete grains, and lean proteins to your meals. Opt for low-sodium options and restrict your intake of processed food, which may be excessive in sodium and threatening components.

To get you started out for your adventure to kidney renewal, we have got protected a few meal making plans guidelines and recipes in this bankruptcy. These recipes are designed to be kidney-first-class, incorporating materials that nourish and assist your kidneys. From colourful salads with a mixture of leafy vegetables and berries to hearty salmon dishes pro with herbs and spices, these recipes aren't handiest delicious however furthermore promote your kidney's health and properly-being.

Making slow dietary adjustments is important to improving kidney characteristic. Start through frequently decreasing your intake of processed components excessive in sodium and dangerous fat. Instead, replace them with nutrient-dense alternatives like sparkling give up end result and veggies. Experiment with new flavors and cooking strategies to make your meals interesting and exciting. Remember, small modifications over the years can reason huge consequences.

By incorporating nutrient-rich substances into your healthy eating plan, you take a proactive approach to assist kidney health and promote renewal. In the subsequent sections of this financial ruin, we can find out mindfulness techniques and herbal treatments that in addition complement your holistic technique to kidney renewal. Together, vitamins, mindfulness, and herbal remedies offer a complete solution for nurturing your kidneys and reaching nice health and electricity.

3. A Holistic Approach to Kidney Renewal: Combining Nutrition, Mindfulness, and Herbal Remedies

Mindfulness Techniques for Optimal Stress Reduction and Kidney Renewal

Stress has a profound effect on our number one well-being, in conjunction with the fitness of our kidneys. When we experience chronic strain, our our bodies release pressure hormones which can bring about contamination and progressed blood stress, each of that could negatively have an effect on kidney characteristic. Therefore, it is important to encompass mindfulness strategies into our every day bodily games to lessen strain and sell rest, in the end supporting kidney renewal.

One effective approach for lowering strain and cultivating mindfulness is meditation. Find a quiet and comfortable area wherein you may sit down or lie down. Close your eyes and recognition your interest for your breath. Notice the feeling of the breath entering into and leaving your frame. Allow any mind or distractions to simply skip by means of without judgment, lightly bringing your hobby decrease again to the breath whenever. Start with only a few minutes an afternoon and little by little growth the duration as you turn out to be greater snug. Regular meditation practice can help calm the mind, alleviate pressure, and create a feel of internal peace that helps kidney health.

Deep respiratory sporting sports are every other effective device for managing stress and promoting relaxation. One simple approach is diaphragmatic respiratory, additionally referred to as stomach breathing. Find a cushty seated position and place one hand on your chest and the alternative to your belly. Take a slow, deep breath in via your nostril, permitting your stomach to upward push as you fill your lungs with air. Exhale slowly thru your mouth, permitting your belly to fall. Repeat this technique several instances, that specialize within the sensation of your breath and consciously freeing any tension or pressure with each exhale. Deep breathing wearing sports assist activate the parasympathetic worried device, which promotes rest and counteracts the effects of stress on the kidneys.

Visualization is any other powerful tool for lowering strain and selling kidney renewal. Close your eyes and keep in mind a peaceful and serene region, which incorporates a tranquil seaside or a lush wooded location. Engage all of your senses with the aid of visualizing the colors, sounds, and scents of this imaginary sanctuary. Allow your self to genuinely immerse in this highbrow photograph and enjoy a enjoy of calm and quietness washing over you. Visualization can help shift your awareness faraway from stressors and create a pleasant and restoration united states of mind that permits kidney fitness.

Incorporating mindfulness into your each day sporting activities is critical for most suitable stress reduction. Start via placing apart committed time every day for mindfulness practices which includes meditation, deep respiration bodily games, or visualization. You can also infuse mindfulness into everyday sports activities. For instance, at the same time as consuming, make the effort to experience every bite, paying attention to the flavors, textures, and smells of your meals. Engaging in aware movement practices like yoga or tai chi also can help reduce stress and promote popular properly-being. By bringing reputation to the prevailing 2nd and cultivating a revel in of gratitude for the nourishment your frame receives, you can assist kidney renewal on a every day basis.

Chapter 6: Unraveling the Ancient Wisdom

Welcome to Chapter four of "The Healing Power of Indigenous Wisdom: Nurturing Your Kidneys for Optimal Health." In this economic catastrophe, we are able to delve into the historical attention of indigenous recovery ideas for kidney health, drawing upon centuries of expertise and conventional practices that have stood the test of time.

These indigenous restoration concepts offer a holistic method to kidney renewal, recognizing the complex connection a few of the mind, body, feelings, and surroundings. By embracing those principles, we are able to free up the ability for transformative recuperation and restore our kidneys to their herbal state of energy.

Throughout this chapter, we're capable of discover the profound knowledge embedded in indigenous recuperation practices. From using plant-based totally completely treatments to the profound recognize for nature and its resources, indigenous recuperation requirements have lots to offer us on our recovery journey.

One of the important thing factors we are able to find out is the usage of herbal treatments derived from herbs and plants. These treatments non-public wonderful houses with first-rate impacts on kidney fitness, which include assisting to cast off pollutants, reducing contamination, and supporting average kidney feature. By understanding and utilizing those natural treatments, we can take an active position in renewing our kidneys in reality.

Furthermore, the ones indigenous recovery thoughts resoundingly emphasize the importance of respecting and connecting with nature. Through this connection, we tap into the recovery electricity of the earth and its assets, fostering a deep revel in of concord and well being internal ourselves. By unraveling and exploring this historical know-how, we gain precious insights into the basis motives of kidney sickness and discover custom designed techniques for kidney renewal.

Lastly, it's miles essential to take a look at that incorporating indigenous healing standards into our complete kidney care plan can complement conventional medical remedies. By drawing close to our kidney health from multiple angles, we are able to decorate our tremendous properly being and sell stability at some point of our entire being.

We invite you to sign up for us in this enlightening and transformative exploration of indigenous recovery principles for kidney fitness. Throughout this financial break, we're capable of unveil the timeless know-how that lies interior these conventional practices and empower ourselves to loose up the proper capability of our kidneys. Let us embark in this adventure of renewal, as we embody the richness of indigenous recuperation and domesticate colorful kidney health and health.

Why Embracing Indigenous Healing Principles is Crucial for Restoring Your Kidneys

In the a long way flung mountains of a tribal village nestled inner a lush, untouched wooded location, a young woman named Amara positioned herself in a struggle for survival. The verdant landscape served as a backdrop to her warfare, as she wrestled with the weight of continual kidney disorder that had plagued her for years.

Amara's life revolved round normal scientific physician visits, laborious treatments, and debilitating aspect outcomes. Her spirit emerge as slowly withering away, overshadowed via using the developing hopelessness that echoed through her weary soul.

But little did Amara understand that her salvation lay in the ancient healing practices rooted in her non-public indigenous manner of existence. With a mixture of desperation and optimism, she launched right into a journey to unearth the age-vintage know-how that promised a glimmer of renewed preference.

Amongst the annoying whispers of the tribal elders and the mystical rituals echoing through the hallowed depths of the forest, Amara unraveled the historical information of her ancestors. These requirements, deeply tied to the interconnectedness of thoughts-body-emotion harmony, supplied steering towards nurturing her struggling kidneys lower again to health.

Guided via an unyielding dedication, Amara explored the herbal treatments exceeded down through generations. She meticulously collected and organized the culinary herbs bestowed upon her by means of manner of the earth itself—trusty allies on her course to restoration. Through trial and errors, she positioned the inner orchestra of her frame responding to those sacred offerings, as diuretic homes flushed out pollutants and the anti-inflammatory prowess calmed infection internal her frail kidneys.

As Amara drank the elixirs of nature, an intimate bond with the earth customary. She learned to be aware of the symphony of the wooded area, slowly spotting the tough connection among her properly-being and the colourful surroundings round her. The healing energy of the historic knowledge flowed through her veins, sparking existence wherein darkness as quick as dwelled.

Transformation unfurled as the flowers embraced Amara, nurturing her like mild guardians. Bolstered by way of way of the accumulated know-how of her indigenous recovery requirements, Amara approached every day with unshakeable resilience. She let circulate of the continual grip of conventional clinical treatments and embraced a herbal and holistic technique founded on centuries of expertise.

Soon, the as soon as-celestial worry that clouded Amara's spirit commenced to use up. The whispers of native treatments crescendoed into the melodies of real restoration. With every passing day, the oppressive fog lifted, uncovering renewed power and an incredible peace inside Amara's center.

The story of Amara underscores the critical importance of unraveling the historic information of indigenous recuperation thoughts for kidney fitness. In her war towards chronic kidney disease, she discovered the transformative strength of embracing her cultural records, honoring the earth's assets, and fostering concord inner herself. Like Amara, allow the chapters that comply with guide you inside the route of unlocking the secrets and techniques and techniques of self-recovery and locating your very personal course to kidney renewal in this first rate tapestry of ancient focus and cutting-edge technological understanding.

Unraveling the Ancient Wisdom: Exploring Indigenous Healing Principles for Kidney Health

Indigenous restoration ideas were handed down thru generations, harnessing ancient expertise and conventional practices to promote kidney renewal. These time-honored techniques have stood the take a look at of time, providing a holistic technique to attaining maximum useful kidney fitness. In this monetary disaster, we are able to delve into the historic context of indigenous recuperation practices, find out the various recuperation traditions of numerous indigenous cultures, and discover particular practices and rituals which might be useful for kidney fitness.

Throughout data, indigenous organizations spherical the arena have superior unique restoration practices based totally on their deep information of nature and the interconnectedness of all living beings. By reading the ancient context of these practices, we gain perception into their origins and the attention they hold. From the ancient Ayurvedic system of India to the Native American recovery traditions, indigenous healing requirements have usually centered on restoring stability and harmony in the frame.

Each indigenous manner of lifestyles has its very private awesome healing traditions that contribute to kidney health. For example, in traditional Chinese remedy, the kidneys are considered the inspiration of essential energy and play a crucial position in commonplace properly-being. Chinese healers emphasize the significance of nourishing the kidneys thru unique dietary alternatives, acupuncture, and herbal treatments. Similarly, Native American recuperation traditions view the kidneys as a sacred organ associated with emotions and the spirit. Rituals concerning sweat motels and medicinal vegetation are completed to cleanse and rejuvenate the kidneys.

Specific restoration practices and rituals associated with kidney fitness vary amongst indigenous cultures. For instance, in Ayurveda, the exercise of Panchakarma goals to take away pollution from the frame through a aggregate of rubdown, herbal remedies, and nutritional adjustments. Traditional Mayan healers employ the power of plant remedy and spiritual ceremonies to restore balance and electricity to the kidneys. By incorporating the ones practices into your very own life, you can faucet into the ancient know-how of indigenous recuperation necessities and promote kidney renewal.

It is crucial to be aware that indigenous restoration practices are deeply rooted in cultural traditions and want to be approached with apprehend and proper know-how. Before incorporating any particular recovery exercise or ritual into your ordinary, it's far beneficial to are searching for steering from experienced practitioners or elders inside the respective indigenous groups. They can provide treasured insights and ensure that the ones practices are finished in a culturally sensitive and appropriate way.

By unraveling the ancient records of indigenous recovery principles for kidney health, we unencumber a treasure trove of expertise and practices that would bring about profound recovery and renewal. Throughout this chapter, we are able to hold to discover the holistic approach of indigenous recovery, which include the mind-frame connection, the characteristic of feelings, environmental elements, and using natural treatments derived from herbs and flowers. Together, we're able to embark on a adventure of self-discovery and empowerment, tapping into the knowledge of our ancestors to nourish our kidneys and beautify our not unusual fitness and well-being.

Unraveling the Ancient Wisdom: Exploring Indigenous Healing Principles for Kidney Health

The thoughts-body connection plays a crucial feature in selling kidney well-being. Indigenous restoration thoughts apprehend the interconnectedness of our intellectual and physical states, emphasizing that our thoughts and emotions can appreciably impact the health of our kidneys. When we experience pressure, tension, or poor emotions, it may motive imbalances inside our our bodies, potentially affecting our kidney function. On the alternative hand, cultivating excessive high-quality thoughts and emotional properly-being can contribute to kidney renewal and commonplace nicely being.

To promote primary kidney health, it is crucial to nurture your emotional well-being. Practicing mindfulness and stress reduction techniques will allow you to control and release terrible emotions that can be burdening your kidneys. Techniques which incorporates deep respiration sporting events, meditation, and yoga can assist lessen strain ranges, sell relaxation, and restore concord interior your body. By incorporating the ones practices into your every day normal, you may useful resource your kidneys' capability to feature optimally.

In addition to the mind-frame connection, information the environmental elements that impact kidney fitness is essential. Pollution, publicity to pollutants, and negative air great can placed a pressure to your kidneys, doubtlessly principal to kidney damage through the years. It is crucial to be aware of your environment and take critical precautions to decrease your exposure to harmful materials. This can embody the use of herbal cleansing merchandise, preserving proper indoor air wonderful, and keeping off contact with poisonous chemical materials each time viable.

To promote holistic nicely-being and harmony, it is beneficial to include numerous strategies into your manner of existence. Engaging in sports activities that supply you satisfaction and fulfillment can actually effect your emotional well-being and, consequently, your kidney fitness. Surrounding your self with awesome and supportive human beings can also contribute to an traditional sense of nicely-being.

Another trouble of selling holistic well-being is nurturing a reference to nature.

Indigenous healing concepts emphasize the importance of acknowledging the healing energy of the earth and its property. Spending time in nature, whether or not or not or now not it's far taking walks in a park, gardening, or truly sitting through a lake, can help restore balance and sell kidney well-being. By incorporating eco-friendly practices into your each day existence, together with decreasing waste and maintaining assets, you can make contributions to each your personal well-being and that of the planet.

In summary, indigenous recuperation thoughts understand the interconnectedness of the mind, body, emotions, and environment in selling kidney properly-being. By nurturing your emotional nicely-being, know-how the environmental factors that affect kidney health, and incorporating techniques for promoting holistic nicely-being and concord, you may aid your kidneys' capacity to characteristic optimally. Remember to workout mindfulness, reduce strain, decrease exposure to pollution, surround yourself with amazing influences, and connect with nature. By incorporating these concepts into your manner of lifestyles, you could pave the manner for renewed kidney fitness and everyday well-being.

Unraveling the Ancient Wisdom: Exploring Indigenous Healing Principles for Kidney Health

Chapter 7: Medicinal Herbs and Plants

The use of medicinal herbs and flowers has prolonged been a cornerstone of indigenous recovery practices for selling kidney health. These natural remedies own specific houses that may be useful in assisting kidney function, which embody diuretic and anti inflammatory homes. In this phase, we are able to discover a number of the normally used herbs and flora in indigenous healing traditions and their particular applications for commonplace kidney situations.

Specific Plant-Based Remedies for Common Kidney Conditions

1. Dandelion Root (Taraxacum officinale): Known for its diuretic homes, dandelion root has been used for hundreds of years to sell kidney health through increasing urine production and supporting to flush out pollution from the body. It can be consumed as an natural tea or taken in

supplement form. Dandelion root is specifically useful for human beings with fluid retention troubles or mild kidney congestion.

2. Corn Silk (Zea mays): Corn silk refers back to the silky threads determined at the ears of corn. It is famend for its diuretic and anti inflammatory residences, that may help lessen swelling and contamination in the kidneys. Corn silk may be brewed right into a tea or taken in pill shape, imparting alleviation for human beings with urinary tract infections, kidney stones, or cutting-edge day kidney infection.

3. Nettle Leaf (Urtica dioica): Nettle leaf is a powerhouse herb that offers severa blessings for kidney fitness. It acts as a diuretic and permits dispose of extra water and waste from the body. Additionally, nettle leaf has anti inflammatory homes that can aid the

discount of kidney irritation. This herb may be enjoyed as a tea or included into culinary dishes as a nutrient-rich food supply.

Tips for Sourcing and Preparing Herbal Remedies Properly

When sourcing herbs and vegetation for medicinal functions, it's far vital to ensure their quality and protection. Here are a few hints to help you supply and prepare natural remedies well:

1. Choose herbal and sustainably sourced herbs: Opt for natural herbs on every occasion possible to keep away from publicity to insecticides and one-of-a-kind volatile chemical substances. Additionally, pick out herbs which might be sustainably harvested to manual environmental conservation.

2. Consult with a informed practitioner: If you are new to using natural treatments, it

is sensible to speak over with a certified herbalist or healthcare practitioner who can manual you in selecting the right herbs and provide suitable dosage tips based totally completely in your specific desires.

3. Follow proper guidance techniques: Different herbs require remarkable training strategies to extract their medicinal homes efficiently. This may additionally additionally include brewing herbal teas, growing tinctures, or using them in culinary dishes. Follow the encouraged schooling techniques to maximize the advantages of the herbs.

4. Be conscious of capability interactions: Some herbs may additionally additionally have interaction with drug treatments or have contraindications for sure humans. It is important to inform your healthcare business enterprise about any herbs or dietary dietary supplements you are taking to avoid any destructive consequences or

interactions with prescribed medicinal pills.

By incorporating the ones indigenous recovery thoughts into your kidney care plan, you can harness the energy of herbal remedies derived from herbs and plant life to manual kidney fitness. Remember to deliver herbs responsibly, comply with right schooling techniques, and are looking for guidance from knowledgeable practitioners to make sure steady and powerful use. The knowledge of indigenous recuperation practices gives a holistic approach to kidney renewal, promoting stability and strength on your normal well-being.

Unraveling the Ancient Wisdom: Exploring Indigenous Healing Principles for Kidney Health

Understanding and applying indigenous recovery ideas requires a deep appreciate and connection to nature, as those standards are rooted in acknowledging the healing power of the earth and its assets. Spiritual and philosophical ideals form the foundation of indigenous restoration practices, guiding human beings on their course to kidney health and everyday properly-being.

Indigenous cultures have prolonged recognized the interconnectedness of human beings with the natural global. They agree with that the earth and its factors maintain profound facts and recovery houses that may be harnessed to repair balance in the frame. By embracing this notion, you may tap into the widespread assets nature affords to useful resource your kidney fitness.

The importance of connecting to nature can't be emphasised sufficient with reference to promoting kidney well-being. Spending time in nature permits you to recharge and harmonize your strength with the natural rhythms of the earth. Whether it's taking a stroll in a nearby park, sitting thru a flowing river, or clearly tending to your very very very own garden, immersing your self in nature has a profound effect on your everyday well-being, which incorporates kidney health.

5. Reconnecting with Nature: Harnessing the Healing Power of Culinary Herbs and Plants

In this charming bankruptcy, we are capable of delve into the enchanting worldwide of culinary herbs and flora, wherein nature's restoration electricity showcases its actual potential for restoring and rejuvenating our treasured kidneys. We will release the secrets and techniques and strategies in the again of the suitable homes that the ones excellent property very own and the manner they will be harnessed to assist kidney health.

The recuperation homes of culinary herbs and flora are diverse and profound. They maintain the functionality to promote cleansing, lessen contamination, and beautify standard kidney feature. Understanding the right utilization and dosage of those herbal marvels is critical for maximizing their healing benefits while minimizing any ability negative outcomes. By incorporating a colorful array of sparkling and natural herbs and plant life into your every day food plan, you can embark on a journey closer to top-exceptional kidney health and renewal.

Within this bankruptcy, we're capable of discover the enriching international of natural teas, crafted from kidney-supportive herbs consisting of dandelion root, nettle leaf, and uva usa. These delightful concoctions can provide a mild but exquisite boom to kidney detoxification, supplying your body a well-deserved pathway to maximum beneficial functionality.

Beyond the vicinity of culinary herbs lie an series of medicinal vegetation imbued with homes that nourish and restore the kidneys. From the mystical aloe vera to the moderate marshmallow root, those hidden gems maintain the capability to repair balance and energy to our precious kidney organs, immersing us in a sea of well-being.

Moreover, we trust that data is pleasant served even as you can end up self-reliant. That's why we are able to explore no longer notable the healing benefits of those stunning items from nature however also equip you with the capabilities to choose out, broaden, and harvest them. By getting to know the paintings of nurturing our very own herbal treatments, we will honestly take manage of our kidney fitness journey.

Indulge in the wonders of nature's pharmacy as you immerse yourself inside the subsequent captivating financial damage of this enlightening adventure in the direction of colorful kidney health and health. Unlock the transformative ability of culinary herbs and flowers, and witness the effective impact they are capable of preserve on your revitalization technique. Are you organized to embark in this awe-inspiring adventure? The transformative electricity of nature awaits your include.

Chapter 8: Embracing Nature's Bounty

Nestled many of the rolling hills of quiet geographical vicinity, there existed a small, picturesque village. The fragrance of blooming flowers permeated the air, and the rhythm of nature's heartbeat might be felt with every passing breeze. In this tranquil haven, the writer encountered a soul whose journey deeply resonated with the message of this economic smash.

This soul has become Maria, a female whose spirit pondered the luxurious splendor of her surroundings. With a smile that radiated warmth and expertise, Maria carried inner her quiet power that spoke volumes. However, unseen to the out of doors international, the struggle inside her non-public frame changed into a long manner from serene.

Maria had lengthy suffered from kidney sickness, its relentless grip tightening with every passing day. She sought solace inside the pages of infinite medical textbooks, however traditional remedies presented no comfort or lasting recuperation. Her coronary heart ached with the burden of a future full of uncertainty, because the energy she as speedy as held high priced slowly commenced to slip away.

Determined to reclaim her life and discover a solution that eluded her draw near, Maria released right into a quest to release the secrets and techniques of self-healing. It emerge as inside the quiet corners of her village, in which nature impassively carried on its everlasting dance, that the forgotten understanding of culinary herbs and flora softly whispered its soothing melody to her longing soul.

With resolute power of will, Maria started out out experimenting with nature's pharmacy, diving deep into the sector of culinary herbs and their transformative powers. Safely guided with the useful resource of the author's teachings on correct utilization and dosage, Maria fearlessly protected an array of sparkling and herbal wonders into her each day food, savoring each moment of this culinary symphony.

Her kitchen transformed into an alchemist's haven, summoning forth the healing magic bottled inside each herb and plant. The colorful colorings of dandelion root and the smooth encompass of nettle leaf infused her teas, supplying her weary kidneys a far-wanted cleaning. And with the comforting presence of uva america of america, the stronghold of infection that had threatened to crumble her remedy diminished with every soothing sip.

But Maria's journey held extra profound revelations. Pulling lower back the curtain that hid the historic restoration secrets and techniques and strategies, she ventured beyond the limits of culinary herbs and embraced a tapestry of medicinal vegetation. With open fingers, she welcomed the rejuvenating embody of aloe vera, its mild contact breathing new existence into her sick kidneys. Marshmallow root, with its mild healing houses, stood as a beacon of desire amidst the gloom of melancholy, encouraging her damaged organs to heal and renew.

As Maria's sowed seeds of expertise sprouted into hopeful blossoms inside her coronary heart, a newfound self assure bloomed within her soul. Grasping the power that lay at her fingertips, she released right into a adventure of self-sufficiency and healing. As she tended to her very very private herb lawn, Maria sturdy a deep, sacred connection with the pulsating rhythms of nature, for all time intertwining her spirit with the collective heartbeat of the Earth.

With tears of delight portray rivers of gratitude upon her cheeks, Maria emerged victorious from the battleground that when solid a shadow upon her life. Her kidneys, once beleaguered thru ailment and depression, started out out whispering reminiscences of renewal and resilience. This transformative journey had not high-quality transformed her bodily properly-being but polished the hidden additives of her soul.

The tale of Maria stands as a testomony, a shimmering beacon in a sea of doubt, illuminating the direction towards self-restoration and the eternal bond among nature and our private sacred vessel. With the information shared within this economic catastrophe, you may additionally comply with in Maria's glossy footsteps, rediscovering the strength of culinary herbs and vegetation to heal, rejuvenate, and nourish your body from internal. Unleash the limitless abundance equipped patiently internal nature's embody, and step ever within the route of a life of renewed energy and boundless nicely-being.

Reconnecting with Nature: Harnessing the Healing Power of Culinary Herbs and Plants

In this economic disaster, we delve into the area of culinary herbs and vegetation and explore their exceptional recovery homes for the kidneys. These natural wonders had been used for loads of years in conventional medicine to sell cleaning, lessen inflammation, and improve kidney function. By incorporating those herbs and plants into your every day regular, you may launch the secrets and techniques and strategies and techniques of self-healing and nurture your kidneys lower again to fine fitness.

Let's start via exploring a number of the vital element culinary herbs and plants famend for his or her kidney restoration houses. One such herb is parsley, stated for its diuretic outcomes that assist flush out pollutants from the kidneys. Rich in antioxidants, parsley moreover aids in decreasing contamination, selling kidney cell restore, and enhancing normal kidney function. Cilantro, every specific flexible herb, not only provides taste in your dishes however moreover supports kidney health with the beneficial resource of detoxifying heavy metals and decreasing oxidative strain.

Ginger and turmeric, effective spices, are widely recognized for their anti-inflammatory homes. By decreasing infection within the kidneys, those herbs can help alleviate symptoms of kidney disease and manual the recuperation manner. Ginger additionally acts as a herbal diuretic, supporting kidney function and flushing out extra fluid.

But how do those culinary herbs and plant life contribute to kidney fitness on a physiological level? It's all approximately their precise mechanisms of movement. Many of those herbs contain antioxidants, which includes flavonoids and polyphenols, which neutralize dangerous unfastened radicals and guard the kidneys from oxidative harm. Additionally, fantastic herbs own diuretic homes, promoting urine production and helping in the elimination of waste and pollution from the frame.

Scientific studies supports using these herbs and plants for kidney health. Numerous studies have examined the beneficial effects of parsley in decreasing blood strain, enhancing kidney feature, and dealing with the development of kidney ailment. Similarly, cilantro has showed promise in defensive in the direction of kidney harm because of heavy metals.

By incorporating the ones culinary herbs and flowers into your weight-reduction plan, you may harness their restoration powers and deliver your kidneys the assist they want. However, it is vital to understand the proper usage and dosage to maximize their recuperation blessings and avoid any potential damaging results.

To make sure you're the use of those herbs and plant life appropriately and efficaciously, it's miles vital to are in search of for recommendation from a healthcare professional or herbalist. They can provide customized recommendations primarily based absolutely definitely in your common fitness, present clinical conditions, and medication interactions. Incorrect utilization or excessive intake of effective herbs and plant life can also have accidental consequences, so it is continually quality to are looking for professional steerage.

When sourcing clean and herbal herbs and plant life, recollect neighborhood farmers' markets or expand them to your very personal herb lawn. By deciding on entire substances and incorporating a numerous variety of herbs and plant life into your food, you could create balanced, nutrient-wealthy dishes that aid average kidney health.

In the following section, we'll find out the blessings of herbal teas crafted from kidney-supportive herbs like dandelion root, nettle leaf, and uva u.S.. These teas offer a available and thrilling manner to promote kidney cleaning and maximum excellent feature. Stay tuned as we discover the secrets and strategies of making herbal teas for max restoration benefit and study potential contraindications or component effects to be aware about.

Understanding the Correct Usage and Dosage of Culinary Herbs and Plants: Maximizing Therapeutic Benefits and Avoiding Adverse Effects

One of the essential element factors in harnessing the healing energy of culinary herbs and vegetation for kidney health is knowing their accurate usage and dosage. While those herbal remedies can provide superb benefits, it's miles essential to method their intake with care to maximize their recovery effects and avoid any functionality negative reactions.

In this financial destroy, we emphasize the significance of consulting with a healthcare expert or herbalist to decide the correct usage and dosage of herbs and flora in your specific desires. Each individual's health profile is specific, and personalized guidelines endure in thoughts factors together with regular health, present scientific conditions, and capacity interactions with medicinal capsules.

By attempting to find steerage from a licensed expert, you may ensure that you're using culinary herbs and plants in a way this is steady and powerful to your kidney health adventure. Professionals skilled in herbal remedy can offer priceless insights into the homes and functionality dangers associated with advantageous herbs and flowers, assisting you are making informed selections about their incorporation into your each day routine.

It is crucial to take a look at that incorrect usage or excessive consumption of splendid herbs and plant life could have unintended consequences. Some herbs can also engage with medicinal drugs, accentuate their consequences, or purpose unfavourable reactions. For example, herbs like ginger or turmeric might also moreover have blood-thinning houses, which may be difficult in case you are already taking anticoagulant medicinal drugs.

That's why it's far vital to understand the capability risks related to particular herbs and vegetation and the manner they will have an impact to your specific activities. By going for walks carefully with a healthcare expert or herbalist, you could mitigate those risks and ensure that your chosen herbs and plants are supporting your kidney health adventure efficiently.

Furthermore, individualized tips for herb and plant usage undergo in mind your simple health and cutting-edge clinical conditions. For instance, when you have a records of allergic reactions or sensitivities, splendid herbs or vegetation might not be suitable for you. On the opportunity hand, if you have specific underlying situations, like excessive blood stress, there may be herbs or vegetation which may be mainly beneficial or need to be approached with warning.

Chapter 9: Understanding Kidney Health

Kidney fitness and illness is a complex and regularly misunderstood concern remembers. The kidneys are bean-long-hooked up organs placed in the decrease lower lower back, one on every trouble of the spine. They are responsible for filtering waste merchandise out of the blood, regulating the body's water stability and electrolyte levels, and producing hormones that help adjust blood pressure and pink blood cell production.

Kidney infection is a well-known time period that describes any form of harm or ailment that influences the kidneys. It is usually because of each a blockage or a lower in function, which can be because of a desire of things. Common motives of kidney illness embody diabetes, immoderate blood strain, an enlarged prostate, glomerulonephritis, and continual kidney infections.

The signs and symptoms of kidney disease vary counting on the type but can embody fatigue, nausea, vomiting, reduced urge for food, swollen ankles and feet, and blood in the urine. It is important to be aware about those symptoms just so remedy can be pursued as rapid as possible.

Treatment for kidney illness can encompass lifestyle changes which include lowering salt consumption, exercise regularly, and keeping off alcohol and cigarettes. Medications together with ACE inhibitors, angiotensin-receptor blockers, and diuretics can also help manipulate signs and symptoms and signs and symptoms and gradual the progression of the illness. In a few instances, dialysis may be important to clean out waste from the blood.

It is critical to be proactive in understanding kidney fitness and illness and to take steps to maintain kidney feature. This consists of normal visits to the physician for check-united states of america of americaand monitoring, as well as heading off sports that could put a pressure at the kidneys, together with the overuse of painkillers or alcohol. Eating a balanced eating regimen and keeping a wholesome weight also can assist inside the prevention of kidney sickness.

By taking the critical steps to live informed and proactive about kidney fitness and sickness, we are able to help make sure that our kidneys are functioning well and that we're taking the important steps to protect them.

When the kidneys come to be damaged or diseased, it can reason a buildup of waste merchandise inside the body, that may cause quite a few medical troubles. Kidney disorder can be attributable to a choice of factors, inclusive of excessive blood strain, diabetes, infections, and inherited conditions.

When it involves expertise kidney fitness, it's miles essential to recognize the signs and signs and symptoms and signs and symptoms and signs and symptoms of kidney infection. If you revel in any of these symptoms and signs and symptoms, it is important to look your health practitioner right away to determine if kidney disease is present.

In addition to facts the signs and symptoms and symptoms and signs of kidney ailment, it is also crucial to understand the way to keep kidney health. The fine manner to do that is to comply with a wholesome manner of lifestyles. Eating a balanced diet regime and exercising regularly can assist to preserve the kidneys functioning well. Additionally, getting everyday test-u.S.With your physician can assist to seize any early symptoms of kidney sickness.

Finally, it is vital to understand the numerous treatments available for kidney sickness. Depending at the severity of the disorder, treatments can variety from way of existence modifications and pills to dialysis or even kidney transplants. It is critical to artwork carefully together with your medical doctor to determine the excellent direction of motion on your case.

Understanding kidney health is critical for keeping a healthful life. By recognizing the signs and symptoms and signs and symptoms and signs and signs of kidney disorder, following a healthy lifestyle, and getting regular take a look at-united stateswith your medical doctor, you can assist keep your kidneys functioning nicely. If you're ever involved approximately the health of your kidneys, do now not hesitate to speak to your medical doctor.

The Benefits of Kidney Cleanse Juicing

Kidney cleanse juicing is an smooth and herbal way to assist help your kidney fitness. This type of juicing can assist rid your body of pollutants, growth your electricity tiers, and beautify your popular fitness. Juicing can also help to reduce inflammation, decorate digestion, and decrease the chance of developing kidney stones in the destiny.

1. Detoxification: Juicing allows to flush out pollution that increase within the kidneys. This can assist to lessen your chance of kidney stones and wonderful kidney-associated problems. Additionally, consuming sparkling juices can help to reduce inflammation inside the body.

2. Improved Digestion: Juicing can assist to enhance the digestive way via imparting the body with crucial nutrients and

minerals. This can help to reduce bloating and decorate traditional digestion.

3. Boosted Immunity: Juicing can help to strengthen your immune system through providing your frame with antioxidants and other crucial nutrients. This can help to reduce your hazard of infection and infection.

4. Increased Energy: Juicing can assist to boom your electricity ranges. This permit you to to live active and alert throughout the day.

5. Improved Nutrient Absorption: Juicing can assist to decorate your body's functionality to take in essential nutrients. This can assist to reduce the threat of nutrient deficiencies and distinct health troubles.

6. Reduced Inflammation: Juicing can help to lessen inflammation within the body. This can help to reduce the risk of growing

persistent illnesses together with arthritis and diabetes.

7. Improved Mood: Juicing can help to enhance your temper with the useful resource of imparting your body with vital vitamins and minerals. This can help to lessen pressure and tension.

8. Improved Kidney Health: Juicing can assist to decorate your kidney health with the aid of the use of flushing out pollution and supplying your frame with important nutrients. This can help to lessen your risk of developing kidney stones and particular kidney-related troubles.

9. Reduced Blood Pressure: Juicing can assist to reduce your blood pressure. This can help to lessen your chance of developing heart sickness and stroke.

10. Weight Loss: Juicing can help to sell weight loss via the use of imparting your frame with critical nutrients and minerals.

Additionally, eating smooth juices can assist to reduce your calorie intake.

In addition to the ones advantages,

eleven. Improved Skin Health: Juicing can help to beautify your pores and pores and skin fitness by means of using imparting your frame with vital vitamins and minerals. This can assist to reduce pimples, wrinkles, and other pores and pores and pores and skin-related problems.

12. Improved Mental Health: Juicing can assist to beautify your intellectual health thru providing your body with essential nutrients and minerals. This can assist to reduce strain and anxiety, similarly to decorate your acquainted highbrow properly-being.

By ingesting sparkling juices often, you can assist to useful resource your everyday health and properly-being. Juicing can help to detoxify your body, lessen inflammation, beautify your digestion, growth your energy stages, and decrease your threat of growing continual illnesses.

With kidney cleanse juicing, you may enjoy a majority of those outstanding advantages and greater.

Getting Started With Kidney Cleanse Juicing

Congratulations on taking step one towards a greater wholesome you by means of way of identifying to get began with a kidney cleanse juicing! Juicing is a awesome manner to detoxify your frame and assist cleanse your kidneys. The kidneys are bean-shaped organs located near the center of your decrease back, in reality under the rib cage. They are responsible for filtering waste, pollutants, and extra fluids from the body.

When you cleanse your kidneys with juicing, you are basically giving your body a mini "reset" in order that it is able to characteristic properly. Juicing permits to flush out pollutants and impurities from the frame, allowing your kidneys to work more effectively. Additionally, the vitamins, minerals, and antioxidants placed in sparkling fruit and vegetable juices can assist to guide normal kidney fitness.

To get began with a kidney cleanse juicing, the first step is to set up a smooth juice recipe. Start through method of selecting some of your desired give up end result and veggies which can be incredible for kidney health. Some awesome alternatives include apples, carrots, beets, celery, cucumber, ginger, and lemon. Make high fine to select out herbal produce every time feasible.

Next, you'll want to determine how lots juice you'd want to make. It's incredible first of all a small amount and increase the amount over the years. Also, hold in thoughts that it's far important to drink the juice proper away after making it, because the nutrients will begin to interrupt down if left sitting for too prolonged.

Finally, you'll need to buy a juicer. There are many different types and types available, so do your studies to discover one that suits your desires. Some of the greater well-known models are centrifugal juicers, masticating juicers, and bloodless-press juicers.

When you've got the whole lot you need, you're organized to get started out! Begin by using washing your produce and reducing it into small portions with a purpose to suit into your juicer. Then, slowly feed the produce into the juicer and accumulate the juice in a pitcher or field. Once you've made your juice, drink it right now for the high-quality results.

Kidney cleanse juicing is an high-quality way to promote everyday health and nicely-being. It can help to flush out pollutants, useful resource kidney fitness, and provide your frame with a boost of vitamins, minerals, and antioxidants. So, in case you're equipped to get commenced out, grasp your juicer and get juicing!

THE BASICS OF KIDNEY CLEANSE JUICING

Kidney cleanse juicing is a form of weight loss plan and way of life alternate that could help to decorate the health of your kidneys. It entails ingesting high quality juices and components which can be particularly designed to assist cleanse and detoxify your kidneys.

The important purpose of kidney cleanse juicing is to help flush out pollutants from your body and growth your simple health and properly-being. This is finished with the aid of ingesting juices which might be rich in vitamins and minerals, as well as distinctive cleaning dealers.

One of the most famous juices for kidney cleanse juicing is lemon juice. This juice is wealthy in diet C, which helps to flush out pollutants out of your frame and permits keep your kidneys healthful. Other beneficial juices encompass apple juice, cranberry juice, and grapefruit juice.

When it includes kidney cleanse juicing, it is critical to select herbal, glowing juices every time feasible. This will ensure which you have grow to be the nice incredible of vitamins and that your body is getting all of the nutrients it desires.

In addition to ingesting juices, you need to moreover increase your intake of water. This will assist to flush out pollutants from your body, further to preserve your kidneys functioning properly.

It is also vital to growth your intake of give up stop result and greens while you're doing a kidney cleanse. Fruits and vegetables are rich in fiber, which permits to maintain your kidneys functioning optimally.

Finally, it is important to keep away from processed food and drink while you're on a kidney cleanse. These forms of components aren't useful in your frame and may make your kidneys artwork more difficult, principal to in addition headaches.

By following the recommendations noted above, you can ensure that you have grow to be all the vitamins and cleansing that include kidney cleanse juicing. Doing this could will will let you enhance your fitness and everyday properly-being.

In addition, it's far recommended to talk on your physician earlier than beginning a kidney cleanse, as they are capable of offer you with custom designed recommendation and ensure that you are doing it effectively.

Chapter 10: Understanding Juicing Ingredients for Kidney Health

If you're inquisitive about enhancing your kidney health, juicing may be a splendid alternative for you. Juicing is a extremely good way to get the nutrients, minerals, and antioxidants you want to manual your kidneys and their everyday functioning. It can also help to flush out pollutants and waste merchandise that may constructing up inside the frame and harm your health.

When juicing for kidney health, it's crucial to understand which elements are superb for your kidneys. First, you'll want to pick out out end result and veggies which might be immoderate in vitamins and minerals, together with apples, oranges, kale, carrots, and beets. These are all terrific property of vitamins that useful resource kidney health.

You ought to also look for additives which are excessive in antioxidants, collectively with blueberries, cranberries, and blackberries. These can assist to lessen contamination within the body, which could help to protect the kidneys from damage and sickness.

In addition to culmination and vegetables, you can additionally want to encompass herbs and spices in your juices. Some of the splendid herbs and spices for kidney fitness encompass ginger, turmeric, and cayenne pepper. These can assist to lessen contamination and help to flush out pollutants from the frame.

Finally, it's vital to apprehend of the amount of sugar you upload in your juices. Excess sugar can positioned a strain in your kidneys, so try to restrict the quantity of added sugar you encompass on your juice. Instead, strive which encompass some drops of honey or a few sparkling fruit to sweeten your juice manifestly.

By expertise which substances are exceptional on your kidneys, you could ensure that your juicing regular is assisting you to achieve most suitable fitness and wellness. Juicing may be a wonderful manner to get the nutrients, minerals, and antioxidants you need to stay healthy and manual your kidneys.

ESSENTIAL INGREDIENTS FOR KIDNEY CLEANSE JUICING

To make sure that your kidneys are functioning well, it's far essential to include crucial additives on your weight loss program to help cleanse and detoxify your kidneys. These crucial components can range from precise foods to herbal dietary dietary supplements and juices and can assist beautify kidney fitness. Some of these embody;

1. Beetroot: Beetroot is rich in antioxidants, which include vitamins C,

nitrates, and betalains, that could assist help kidney fitness. It may also additionally furthermore help reduce inflammation, beautify blood flow, and decrease oxidative pressure within the kidneys.

2. Carrot: Carrots are wealthy in beta-carotene, which permits to reduce infection and guard the kidneys from oxidative damage. Additionally, carrots are excessive in fiber, which helps to lessen high cholesterol levels, this is related to kidney harm.

3. Celery: Celery is rich in antioxidants, which embody vitamins C, which could help lessen inflammation and boost kidney fitness. It additionally carries diuretic houses that could assist flush out pollutants from the body, this is crucial for kidney fitness.

four. Berries: Berries are immoderate in antioxidants, inclusive of anthocyanins and polyphenols, that may assist shield the kidneys from oxidative pressure. Additionally, berries are wealthy in fiber, that may help lessen excessive levels of cholesterol, which might be linked to kidney harm.

5. Greens: Leafy greens, together with spinach, kale, and collards, are excessive in antioxidants and fiber, which can assist reduce infection and guard the kidneys from damage. Additionally, vegetables are immoderate in chlorophyll, which could assist detoxify the frame and assist kidney health.

6. Ginger: Ginger is a powerful anti-inflammatory and may help lessen irritation inside the kidneys. Additionally, ginger can assist reduce oxidative strain, this is related to kidney harm.

7. Apple Cider Vinegar: Apple cider vinegar is wealthy in antioxidants, together with

acetic acid and polyphenols, that may assist shield the kidneys from oxidative stress. Additionally, it could assist lessen inflammation and excessive cholesterol levels, which may be both related to kidney harm.

eight. Turmeric: Turmeric is a effective anti inflammatory, and might assist reduce contamination within the kidneys and guard them from oxidative damage. Additionally, turmeric can help lessen immoderate levels of cholesterol, which is probably associated with kidney harm.

9. Lemon: Lemons are immoderate in weight loss program C and antioxidants, that can help lessen infection and guard the kidneys from oxidative strain. Additionally, lemons are immoderate in fiber, that may help reduce immoderate cholesterol levels, it clearly is related to kidney harm.

10. Watermelon: Watermelon is excessive in antioxidants, inclusive of lycopene, that may help protect the kidneys from oxidative pressure. Additionally, it is able to assist lessen inflammation and excessive cholesterol levels, which can be every related to kidney damage.

eleven. Parsley: Parsley is rich in antioxidants, together with eating regimen C, that could assist reduce contamination and guard the kidneys from oxidative damage. Additionally, parsley is a diuretic, which can help flush out pollutants from the body, this is critical for kidney fitness.

12. Coconut Water: Coconut water is wealthy in electrolytes and potassium, that can assist lessen contamination and protect the kidneys from harm. Additionally, it could assist lessen high cholesterol levels, which might be associated with kidney harm.

thirteen. Cucumber: Cucumbers are a diuretic, that could help flush out pollution from the frame, that is important for kidney health. Additionally, cucumbers are high in antioxidants, together with nutrients C, that could assist reduce irritation and shield the kidneys from oxidative harm.

14. Garlic: Garlic is a powerful anti inflammatory, and can assist lessen contamination inside the kidneys and guard them from oxidative harm. Additionally, garlic can help reduce excessive levels of cholesterol, which can be related to kidney harm.

15. Avocado: Avocados are rich in antioxidants and fiber, which can help reduce infection and shield the kidneys from oxidative damage. Additionally, avocados are excessive in potassium, that could assist lessen immoderate cholesterol

levels, which may be linked to kidney damage.

16. Water: Water is critical for keeping the kidneys healthy and it allows flush out pollution from the frame, it really is essential for kidney fitness. Additionally, water can help reduce contamination, enhance blood glide, and decrease oxidative stress within the kidneys.

17. Olive Oil: Olive oil is rich in antioxidants, which includes polyphenols, which can help defend the kidneys from oxidative damage. Additionally, it is able to assist lessen irritation and excessive levels of cholesterol, which might be both linked to kidney harm.

18. Green Tea: Green tea is wealthy in antioxidants, at the facet of catechins, which can assist lessen infection and guard the kidneys from oxidative damage. Additionally, it could assist lessen high

levels of cholesterol, which may be connected to kidney harm.

19. Parsnips: Parsnips are immoderate in fiber, that can help reduce high levels of cholesterol, which may be related to kidney damage. Additionally, parsnips are rich in antioxidants, which includes diet C, which can assist lessen irritation and protect the kidneys from oxidative harm.

20. Cranberry Juice: Cranberry juice is rich in antioxidants, which incorporates anthocyanins, that would assist lessen infection and shield the kidneys from oxidative harm. Additionally, it can assist lessen excessive cholesterol levels, which can be related to kidney harm.

21. Artichoke: Artichokes are rich in antioxidants, along with caffeic acid, that can help lessen infection and defend the kidneys from oxidative harm. Additionally, artichokes are excessive in fiber, that

would help reduce excessive levels of cholesterol, which might be related to kidney damage.

22. Pumpkin: Pumpkin is wealthy in antioxidants, collectively with beta-carotene and nutrition C, that might help lessen infection and guard the kidneys from oxidative damage. Additionally, it could assist lessen excessive levels of cholesterol, which may be connected to kidney damage.

23. Papaya: Papaya is excessive in antioxidants, together with beta-carotene and food regimen C, that could help lessen infection and protect the kidneys from oxidative harm. Additionally, it can help reduce immoderate levels of cholesterol, which might be linked to kidney damage.

24. Broccoli: Broccoli is immoderate in antioxidants, which includes food plan C and sulforaphane, which could help

reduce infection and guard the kidneys from oxidative damage. Additionally, it can help reduce immoderate cholesterol levels, which can be related to kidney damage.

25. Tomatoes: Tomatoes are excessive in antioxidants, together with lycopene and nutrients C, which could assist reduce infection and shield the kidneys from oxidative damage. Additionally, it can assist reduce excessive levels of cholesterol, which may be related to kidney harm.

26. Pomegranate: Pomegranates are immoderate in antioxidants, collectively with punicalagin and ellagic acid, that can assist reduce infection and shield the kidneys from oxidative harm.

Essential Juicing Techniques

Juicing has grow to be increasingly more famous in modern-day years as a manner to get all of the nutrients one desires at the identical time as keeping off the hassle of having geared up a meal. While it can appear to be a easy approach, there are pretty some critical juicing techniques that permit you to get the maximum out of your enjoy.

The first step is to select the proper substances. You want to select out out sparkling, ripe end result and greens which is probably in season. This will assist guarantee which you get the most nutrients out of your juice. Also, make certain to smooth and peel any produce that goals it.

Next, you may need to decide what form of juicer you need to apply. There are hundreds of sorts to be had, from favored centrifugal juicers to extra superior masticating juicers. Generally, masticating juicers provide better quality juice and are higher for leafy veggies.

When you're ready to begin juicing, it is crucial to cut the produce into small portions. This will allow the juicer to extract greater juice from the produce, resulting in a extra nutrient-dense drink. It is likewise vital to change amongst difficult and tender quit result and greens to ensure that the juicer can address the product without getting clogged.

TIPS FOR CRAFTING DELICIOUS KIDNEY CLEANSE JUICES

When it entails crafting scrumptious kidney cleanse juices, it's far essential to understand the basics of what your frame wants to sell wholesome kidney function. The kidneys are an vital organ within the body and play a characteristic inside the filtration and elimination of waste products from the bloodstream. Juicing can assist aid the kidneys with the aid of way of manner of imparting essential vitamins and minerals that can be missing within the diet, further to supporting to flush out pollution and waste products. To get the most out of your kidney cleanse juices, right here are some pointers to keep in thoughts.

1. Balance your substances: Make tremendous your juice consists of a balance of give up cease end result, veggies, herbs, and spices. This will make certain which you get the most out of the vitamins and blessings of the additives.

2. Choose the proper end result and vegetables: Fruits and vegetables which is probably high in antioxidants, nutrients, and minerals are important for kidney health. Some of the exceptional factors for a kidney cleanse juice embody beets, celery, ginger, apples, cucumbers, carrots, garlic, spinach, and mint.

3. Get revolutionary with recipes: Experimenting with specific recipes is a

superb manner to make certain your juice is tasty and nutritious. Try such as some tablespoons of superfood powders to decorate the nutritional rate of your juice.

4. Drink your juice smooth: Freshly made juice is continuously excellent, because it will provide the maximum nutrients and benefits. If you plan on consuming your juice later, shop it in a sealed field in the fridge and drink it internal more than one days.

five. Add healthful fats: Healthy fats help to take in the vitamins and minerals in your juice, so don't forget including some flaxseed oil, coconut oil, or avocado for your juice.

6. Drink plenty of water: Drinking plenty of water within the route of the day is critical for correct kidney function.

7. Avoid along with too much sugar: Too lots sugar may be terrible to kidney health,

so try and limit the amount of candy culmination you add for your juices.

8. Listen for your body: If you experience any bad aspect results from your juices, which incorporate nausea or headaches, prevent ingesting them and are trying to find advice out of your health practitioner.

By following those hints, you need with the intention to craft delicious and nutritious kidney cleanse juices a superb way to help to assist your kidney fitness. Enjoy!

Chapter 11: Kidney Cleanse Juicing Recipes

1. Cucumber and Celery Juice:

Ingredients:

2 cucumbers

2 stalks of celery

2 tablespoons of freshly compressed lemon juice

2 cups of water

Method of Preparation:

Peel and reduce the cucumbers into small portions.

Cut the celery into small quantities.

Place the cucumbers, celery, lemon juice, and water in a blender or meals processor and mix until clean.

Pour the juice into a pitcher and enjoy.

Storage:

Store any final juice in an hermetic area in the refrigerator for up to 3 days.

2. Beet and Carrot Juice:

Ingredients:

2 beets

2 carrots

2 tablespoons of freshly compressed lemon juice

2 cups of water

Method of Preparation:

Peel and reduce the beets and carrots into small pieces.

Place the beets, carrots, lemon juice, and water in a blender or food processor and blend till easy.

Pour the juice into a pitcher and enjoy.

Storage:

Store any final juice in an airtight place inside the fridge for up to 3 days.

three. Spinach and Apple Juice:

Ingredients:

2 cups of spinach

2 apples

2 tablespoons of freshly compressed lemon juice

2 cups of water

Method of Preparation:

Wash and chop the spinach.

Core and decrease the apples into little pieces.

Place the spinach, apples, lemon juice, and water in a blender or meals processor and blend until clean.

Pour the juice into a pitcher and experience.

Storage:

Store any ultimate juice in an hermetic field within the refrigerator for up to a few days.

4. Grapefruit and Carrot Juice:

Ingredients:

2 grapefruits

2 carrots

2 tablespoons of freshly compressed lemon juice

2 cups of water

Method of Preparation:

Peel and reduce the grapefruits into small pieces.

Peel and decrease the carrots into little portions.

Place the grapefruits, carrots, lemon juice, and water in a blender or meals processor and mix till clean.

Pour the juice into a tumbler and enjoy.

Storage:

Store any ultimate juice in an hermetic field inside the refrigerator for up to 3 days.

five. Parsley and Apple Juice:

Ingredients:

2 cups of parsley

2 apples

2 tablespoons of freshly compressed lemon juice

2 cups of water

Method of Preparation:

Wash and chop the parsley.

Core and decrease the apples into little portions.

Place the parsley, apples, lemon juice, and water in a blender or meals processor and blend until easy.

Pour the juice into a pitcher and enjoy.

Storage:

Store any closing juice in an airtight field inside the fridge for up to 3 days.

6. Kale and Cucumber Juice:

Ingredients:

2 cups of kale

2 cucumbers

2 tablespoons of freshly compressed lemon juice

2 cups of water

Method of Preparation:

Wash and chop the kale.

Peel and reduce the cucumbers into small portions.

Place the kale, cucumbers, lemon juice, and water in a blender or food processor and mix till easy.

Pour the juice into a tumbler and experience.

Storage:

Store any last juice in an airtight box inside the refrigerator for up to three days.

7. Broccoli and Pear Juice:

Ingredients:

2 cups of broccoli

2 pears

2 tablespoons of freshly compressed lemon juice

2 cups of water

Method of Preparation:

Wash and chop the broccoli.

Core and reduce the pears into small quantities.

Place the broccoli, pears, lemon juice, and water in a blender or meals processor and blend until smooth.

Pour the juice into a glass and enjoy.

Storage:

Store any final juice in an hermetic concern within the refrigerator for up to 3 days.

eight. Celery and Avocado Juice:

Ingredients:

2 stalks of celery

1 avocado

2 tablespoons of freshly compressed lemon juice

2 cups of water

Method of Preparation:

Cut the celery into small portions.

Peel and pit the avocado and chop it into little quantities.

Place the celery, avocado, lemon juice, and water in a blender or food processor and mix till smooth.

Pour the juice into a tumbler and revel in.

Storage:

Store any closing juice in an hermetic field inside the refrigerator for up to a few days.

nine. Banana and Spinach Juice:

Ingredients:

1 banana

2 cups of spinach

2 tablespoons of freshly compressed lemon juice

2 cups of water

Method of Preparation:

Peel and decrease the banana into little pieces.

Wash and chop the spinach.

Place the banana, spinach, lemon juice, and water in a blender or food processor and mix till clean.

Pour the juice into a pitcher and experience.

Storage:

Store any final juice in an hermetic field inside the fridge for up to 3 days.

10. Kiwi and Carrot Juice:

Ingredients:

2 kiwis

2 carrots

2 tablespoons of freshly compressed lemon juice

2 cups of water

Method of Preparation:

Peel and decrease the kiwis into little pieces.

Peel and decrease the carrots into small quantities.

Place the kiwis, carrots, lemon juice, and water in a blender or meals processor and blend till smooth.

Pour the juice into a glass and experience.

Storage:

Store any closing juice in an airtight subject inside the refrigerator for up to three days.

11. Mango and Parsley Juice:

Ingredients:

1 mango

2 cups of parsley

2 tablespoons of freshly compressed lemon juice

2 cups of water

Method of Preparation:

Peel and reduce the mango into little quantities.

Wash and chop the parsley.

Place the mango, parsley, lemon juice, and water in a blender or meals processor and blend until smooth.

Pour the juice into a pitcher and enjoy.

Storage:

Store any ultimate juice in an airtight subject inside the refrigerator for up to 3 days.

12. Pineapple and Cucumber Juice:

Ingredients:

1 pineapple

2 cucumbers

2 tablespoons of freshly compressed lemon juice

2 cups of water

Method of Preparation:

Peel, center, and decrease the pineapple into little quantities.

Peel and decrease the cucumbers into small pieces.

Place the pineapple, cucumbers, lemon juice, and water in a blender or meals processor and blend until clean.

Pour the juice into a tumbler and revel in.

Storage:

Store any final juice in an hermetic discipline inside the refrigerator for up to 3 days.

thirteen. Orange and Broccoli Juice:

Ingredients:

2 oranges

2 cups of broccoli

2 tablespoons of freshly compressed lemon juice

2 cups of water

Method of Preparation:

Peel and cut the oranges into small portions.

Wash and chop the broccoli.

Place the oranges, broccoli, lemon juice, and water in a blender or meals processor and blend till easy.

Pour the juice into a pitcher and enjoy.

Storage:

Store any final juice in an airtight container inside the refrigerator for up to 3 days.

14. Beet and Apple Juice:

Ingredients:

2 beets

2 apples

2 tablespoons of freshly compressed lemon juice

2 cups of water

Method of Preparation:

Peel and reduce the beets into little quantities.

Core and decrease the apples into little quantities.

Place the beets, apples, lemon juice, and water in a blender or meals processor and mix until easy.

Pour the juice into a pitcher and experience.

Storage:

Store any remaining juice in an airtight container in the fridge for up to a few days.

15. Avocado and Carrot Juice:

Ingredients:

1 avocado

2 carrots

2 tablespoons of freshly compressed lemon juice

2 cups of water

Method of Preparation:

Peel and pit the avocado and reduce it into little portions.

Peel and decrease the carrots into little quantities.

Place the avocado, carrots, lemon juice, and water in a blender or food processor and mix until smooth.

Pour the juice into a glass and experience.

Storage:

Store any closing juice in an hermetic field in the refrigerator for up to 3 days.

16. Pear and Celery Juice:

Ingredients:

2 pears

2 stalks of celery

2 tablespoons of freshly compressed lemon juice

2 cups of water

Method of Preparation:

Core and decrease the pears into little portions.

Cut the celery into small portions.

Place the pears, celery, lemon juice, and water in a blender or meals processor and blend until smooth.

Pour the juice into a pitcher and revel in it.

Storage:

Store any last juice in an hermetic area inside the refrigerator for up to three days.

17. Carrot and Banana Juice:

Ingredients:

2 carrots

1 banana

2 tablespoons of freshly compressed lemon juice

2 cups of water

Method of Preparation:

Peel and reduce the carrots into little quantities.

Peel and reduce the banana into little portions.

Place the carrots, banana, lemon juice, and water in a blender or food processor and blend until clean.

Pour the juice into a glass and revel in.

Storage:

Store any very last juice in an hermetic field within the fridge for up to a few days.

18. Kale and Orange Juice:

Ingredients:

2 cups of kale

2 oranges

2 tablespoons of freshly squeezed lemon juice

2 cups of water

Method of Preparation:

Wash and chop the kale.

Peel and reduce the oranges into small quantities.

Place the kale, oranges, lemon juice, and water in a blender or meals processor and blend till smooth.

Pour the juice into a tumbler and revel in.

Storage:

Store any ultimate juice in an hermetic issue in the refrigerator for up to a few days.

19. Parsley and Grapefruit Juice:

Ingredients:

2 cups of parsley

2 grapefruits

2 tablespoons of freshly compressed lemon juice

2 cups of water

Method of Preparation:

Wash and chop the parsley.

Peel and reduce the grapefruits into little portions.

Place the parsley, grapefruits, lemon juice, and water in a blender or food processor and blend till clean.

Pour the juice into a glass and experience.

Storage:

Store any final juice in an airtight discipline in the refrigerator for up to three days.

20. Spinach and Mango Juice:

Ingredients:

2 cups of spinach

1 mango

2 tablespoons of freshly compressed lemon juice

2 cups of water

Method of Preparation:

Wash and chop the spinach.

Peel and cut the mango into small portions.

Place the spinach, mango, lemon juice, and water in a blender or meals processor and mix till clean.

Pour the juice into a tumbler and experience.

Storage:

Store any final juice in an airtight discipline in the refrigerator for up to three days.

21. Banana and Celery Juice:

Ingredients:

1 banana

2 stalks of celery

2 tablespoons of freshly compressed lemon juice

2 cups of water

Method of Preparation:

Peel and cut the banana into small portions.

Cut the celery into small portions.

Place the banana, celery, lemon juice, and water in a blender or meals processor and mix till easy.

Pour the juice into a glass and revel in.

Storage:

Store any very last juice in an airtight field inside the refrigerator for up to a few days.

22. Apple and Avocado Juice:

Ingredients:

2 apples

1 avocado

2 tablespoons of freshly compressed lemon juice

2 cups of water

Method of Preparation:

Core and decrease the apples into little portions.

Peel and pit the avocado and reduce it into little portions.

Place the apples, avocado, lemon juice, and water in a blender or meals processor and mix till easy.

Pour the juice into a pitcher and enjoy.

Storage:

Store any very last juice in an hermetic field inside the refrigerator for up to a few days.

23. Carrot and Kiwi Juice:

Ingredients:

2 carrots

2 kiwis

2 tablespoons of freshly compressed lemon juice

2 cups of water

Method of Preparation:

Peel and decrease the carrots into little pieces.

Peel and decrease the kiwis into little pieces.

Place the carrots, kiwis, lemon juice, and water in a blender or food processor and mix until easy.

Pour the juice into a glass and enjoy.

Storage:

Store any remaining juice in an hermetic container in the refrigerator for up to 3 days.

24. Cucumber and Pineapple Juice:

Ingredients:

2 cucumbers

1 pineapple

2 tablespoons of freshly compressed lemon juice

2 cups of water

Method of Preparation:

Peel and decrease the cucumbers into little quantities.

Peel, middle, and reduce the pineapple into little portions.

Place the cucumbers, pineapple, lemon juice, and water in a blender or food processor and mix till clean.

Pour the juice into a glass and enjoy.

Storage:

Store any remaining juice in an airtight discipline in the fridge for up to three days.

25. Beet and Parsley Juice:

Ingredients:

2 beets

2 cups of parsley

2 tablespoons of freshly compressed lemon juice

2 cups of water

Method of Preparation:

Peel and reduce the beets into little quantities.

Wash and chop the parsley.

Place the beets, parsley, lemon juice, and water in a blender or food processor and blend till smooth.

Pour the juice into a pitcher and experience.

Storage:

Store any final juice in an airtight box within the refrigerator for up to 3 days.

26. Orange and Kale Juice:

Ingredients:

2 oranges

2 cups of kale

2 tablespoons of freshly compressed lemon juice

2 cups of water

Method of Preparation:

Peel and decrease the oranges into little quantities.

Wash and chop the kale.

Place the oranges, kale, lemon juice, and water in a blender or food processor and mix until easy.

Pour the juice into a glass and revel in.

Storage:

Store any last juice in an airtight subject in the fridge for up to 3 days.

27. Avocado and Apple Juice:

Ingredients:

1 avocado

2 apples

2 tablespoons of freshly compressed lemon juice

2 cups of water

Method of Preparation:

Peel and pit the avocado and reduce it into little pieces.

Core and reduce the apples into little quantities.

Place the avocado, apples, lemon juice, and water in a blender or food processor and mix until clean.

Pour the juice into a pitcher and enjoy.

Storage:

Store any final juice in an airtight field within the refrigerator for up to 3 days.

www.ingramcontent.com/pod-product-compliance
Lightning Source LLC
Chambersburg PA
CBHW051726020426
42333CB00014B/1183